# Intermittent FASTING
## FOR WOMEN OVER 50

Feeling Like in Your Fabulous Thirty Again is Doable.
A Beginner's Guide to Start Fasting
With No Lifestyle Changes

Including:
# 30-DAY MEAL PLAN
# 150+ RECIPES
# 7-DAY WORKOUT PLAN

*Christine Bergs*

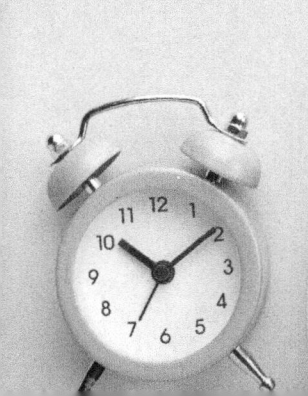

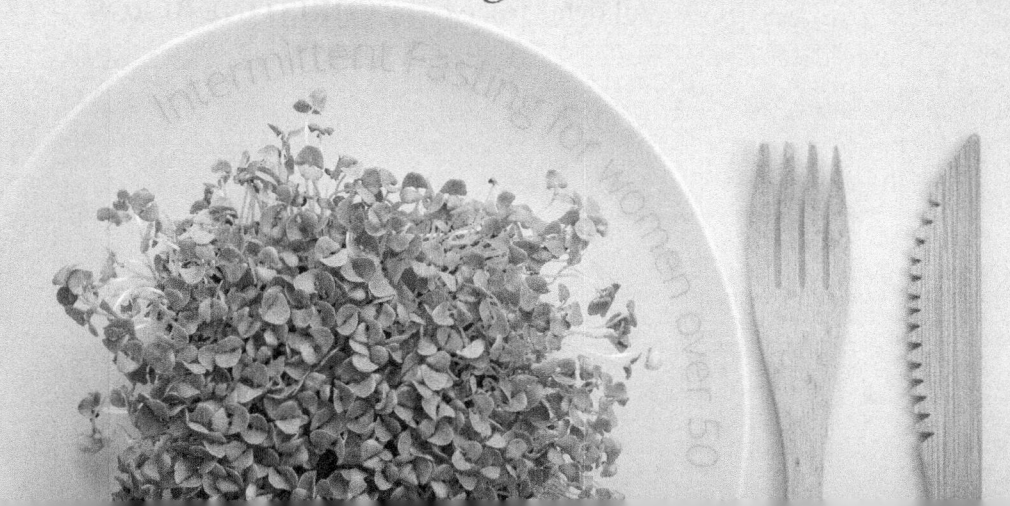

**Copyright ©2021 by CHRISTINE BERGS.**
**All rights reserved.**

No part of this book may be reproduced in any form or by any mechanical means, including information storage and retrieval systems, without permission in writing from the publisher/author, except by a reviewer who may quote passages in a review.

The book is for informational and educational purposes only. Author/publisher will not be held responsible for any damages, monetary loss or reparations that could arise from use of any information contained within the book.

All images, logos, quotes, and trademarks included in this book are subject to use according to trademark and copyright laws of the United States.

Reading of this book constitutes consent agreement to the above requirements.

All rights reserved by **CHRISTINE BERGS**

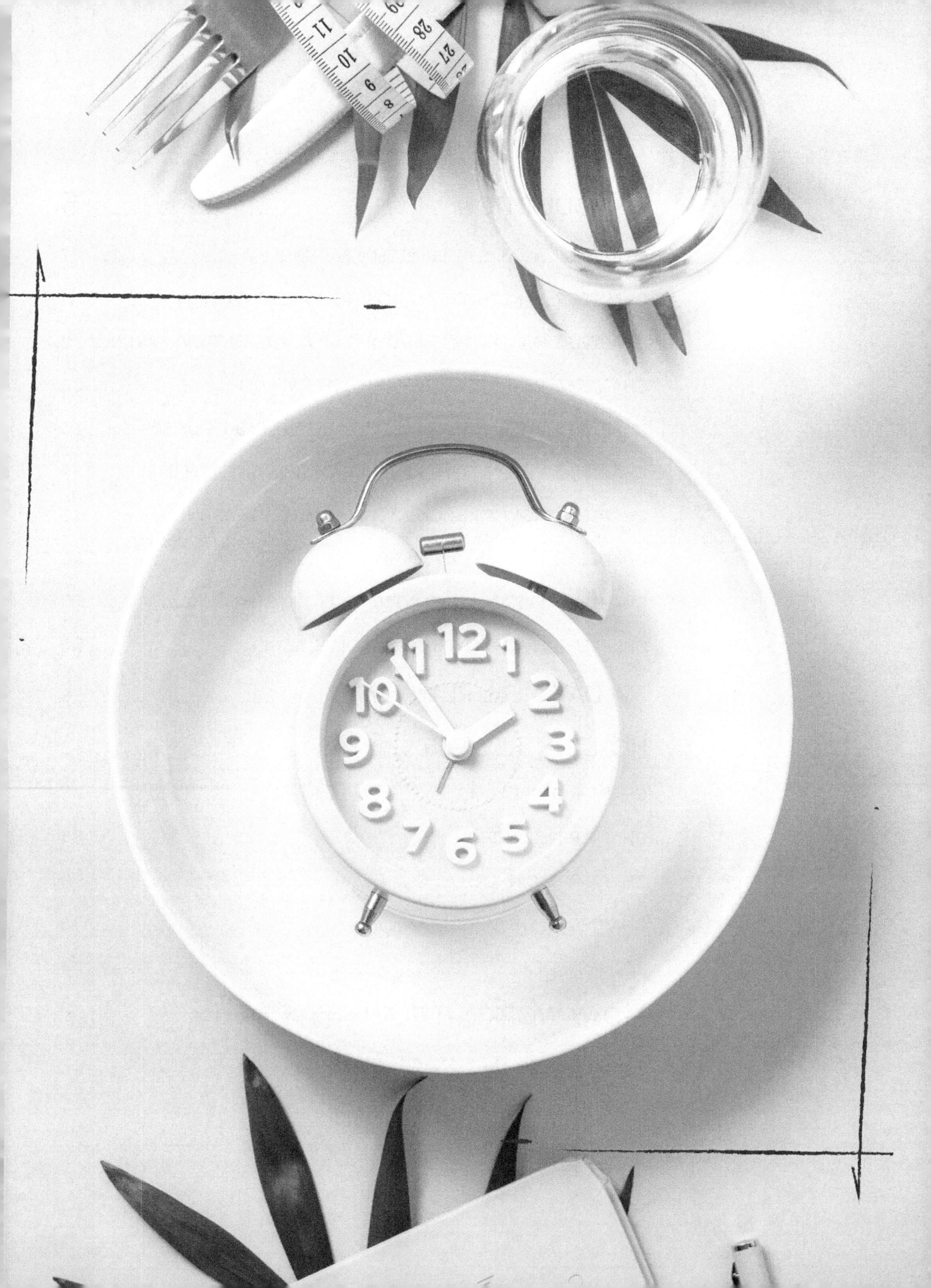

# Table of Contents

INTRODUCTION ................................................................. 5

CHAPTER 1: WHAT IS INTERMITTENT FASTING? ........................ 7

CHAPTER 2: 10 METHODS TO DO INTERMITTENT FASTING ............. 11

CHAPTER 3: FOOD TO EAT AND AVOID ON INTERMITTENT FASTING . 22

CHAPTER 4: BENEFITS OF INTERMITTENT FASTING ..................... 28

CHAPTER 5: INTERMITTENT FASTING AND THE FABULOUS 50s ....... 33

CHAPTER 6: INTERMITTENT FASTING POSSIBLE SIDE EFFECTS ........ 39

CHAPTER 7: HOW TO STICK INTO INTERMITTENT FASTING ............ 43

CHAPTER 8: MISTAKES TO AVOID ........................................ 46

CHAPTER 9: EXERCISE AND INTERMITTENT FASTING ................. 50

CHAPTER 10: FAQ & MYTH TO DISSOLVE ............................... 54

## 30-DAY MEAL PLAN ........................................................ 58

## HEALTHY RECIPES .......................................................... 63

CHAPTER 11: BREAKFAST .................................................. 67

CHAPTER 12: LUNCH ....................................................... 83

CHAPTER 13: DINNER ..................................................... 100

CHAPTER 14: SNACKS ..................................................... 118

RECIPES INDEX ............................................................. 124

## 7-DAY WORKOUT PLAN - BONUS CHAPTER - .......... 127

## CONCLUSION ............................................................. 144

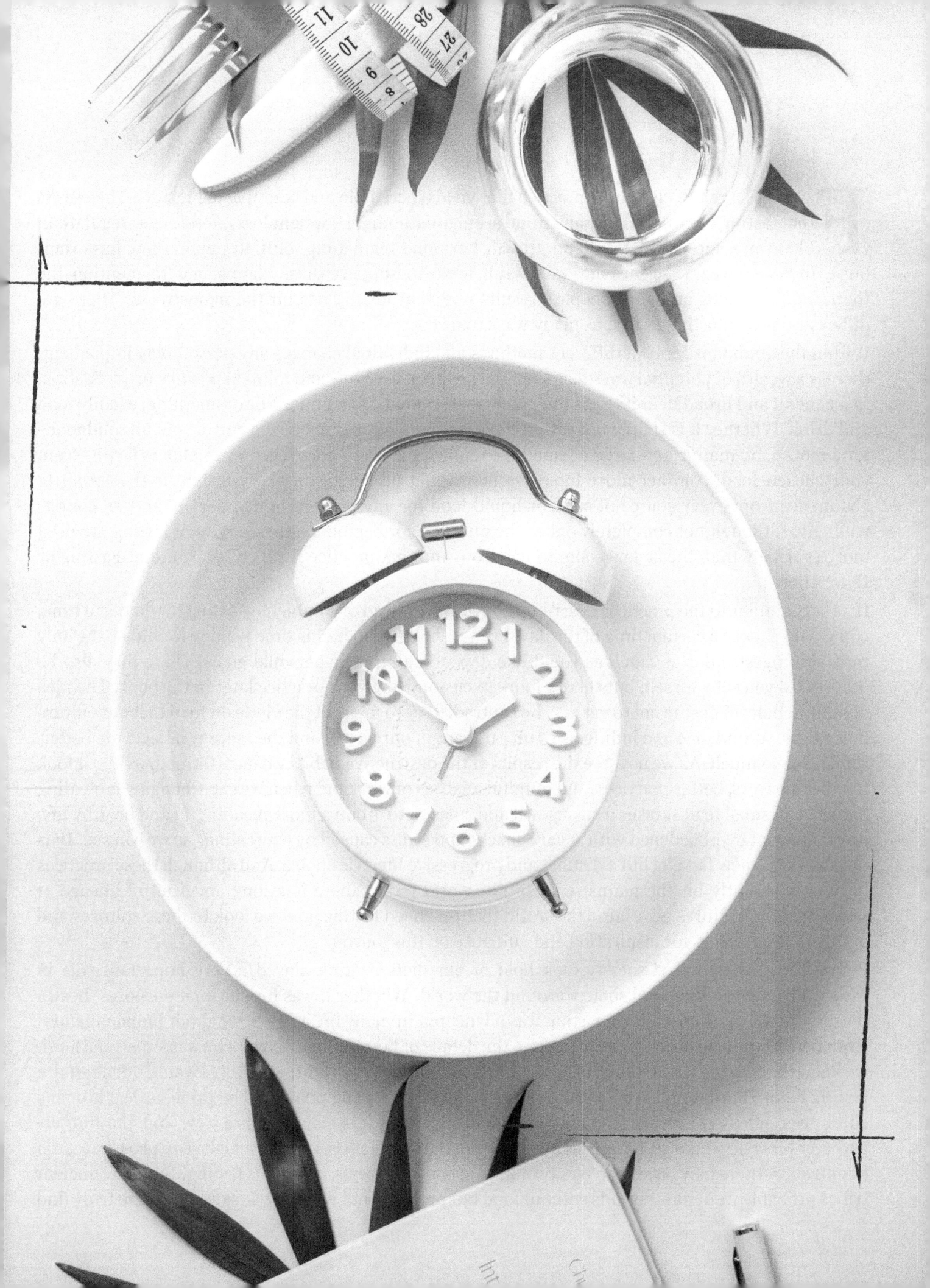

# Introduction

Fasting is a relatively simple practice that yields incredible and complicated results. The effects that fasting has on the body and mind seem unfathomable: weight loss, blood sugar regulation, blood pressure regulation, and growth hormone regulation—only to name a few important ones. In recent years, science has come full force to support these claims, not to mention the thousands of videos online of people's results now that fasting has hit the mainstream. There are different types of fasting as well as many ways to fast.

Within the abundant array of different methods and individual changes any person may implement, there is a wealth of potential ways to impact the health of the body and mind in positive ways. Fasting, in a general and broad definition, is the practice of willingly abstaining from something, usually food and drink. Whether it is simply not eating chocolate for a week or 2 or even cutting out all solid foods for a month, no matter how large or small the impact, the abstinence has on you, that is fasting from your chosen food. Another more intensive fast would be dry fasting. Dry fasting is the complete abstinence from every source of solid or liquid food for any predetermined period, and, of course, willingly. Although not completely out of the question for beginners, these styles of fasting are used more sparingly than the style we aim to focus on, and that practice is called Intermittent Fasting or IF for short.

IF is very similar to the practices described above, but instead of completely fasting for days at a time, you would choose a certain time of the day, say a 12-hour period. This time window would be the only time you ingest foods as much as you'd like depending on your personal goals. There may also be other rules you set yourself, but there's more to customizing your practice later in the book. The idea of intentionally choosing not to eat may be contradictory to many of the views on food that our culture holds dear. Abundance and indulgence run rampant in our world, and the more you have, the better, right? Not so much. As we now see the results of the destructive habits we have formed, we must look to other answers, better practices, and mindful analysis of what and when we eat. Changing our eating habits is no small feat; it takes a strong will and a desire to attain a more meaningful and healthy life, one that is not overburdened with sugary snacks and stress caused by overeating. As we can see, IF is not so much a new fad diet but a distinct and progressive lifestyle choice. And although these practices have only recently hit the mainstream in our world today, there is a long and fruitful lineage of practices from cultures all around the world that practiced fasting, and we look to these cultures and our distant ancestors for inspiration and guidance on this journey.

Before today's fast-paced society took hold of our diets, fasting played a very important role in essentially every culture and society around the world. Whether it was for spiritual purposes, health reasons, or some intense ritual, fasting was a lynchpin in many lifestyles throughout human history. Even before humans had science to explore the details of how our bodies work on a microscopic level, we knew that fasting was a source of good health and wellbeing. Primitive cultures would often require fasting before battles and even as an initiatory milestone during puberty. The prehistorical humans surely weren't as concerned about their weight and appearances as we are now, but the hunter-gatherer lifestyle would seemingly fit nicely within the scope of IF. Wandering place to place in search of nutrients, there may have been plenty of time in between meals, but is this fasting? Sure, the ancient tribes probably went long periods without food but probably not willingly. It's impossible to truly find out what the ancient cultures were thinking and practicing, but here, we see potential caloric restriction that influenced early man in incredible ways, perhaps even influencing the onset of agriculture and settling.

As humans progressed and began settling, we saw a more prominent and definitive practice of fasting. We see all the big hitters in the religious world advocating for it; Jesus Christ, Muhammed, and Buddha all viewed fasting as a purification process. Commonly based on religious grounds, fasting became a practice of sacrifice, giving up something to show a respected God or entity that you were devoted and deserved good graces from powerful beings. The idea of giving up something so precious, which was required to survive, would surely appease the gods. Certainly, as these practices caught on, the humans, religious or not, felt the results of their fasts. Fasting stays a prominent aspect of medicine as the timeline progresses onward into some ancient cultures that we have better historical documentation of.

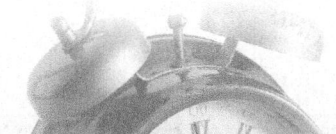

## CHAPTER 1

# What is Intermittent Fasting?

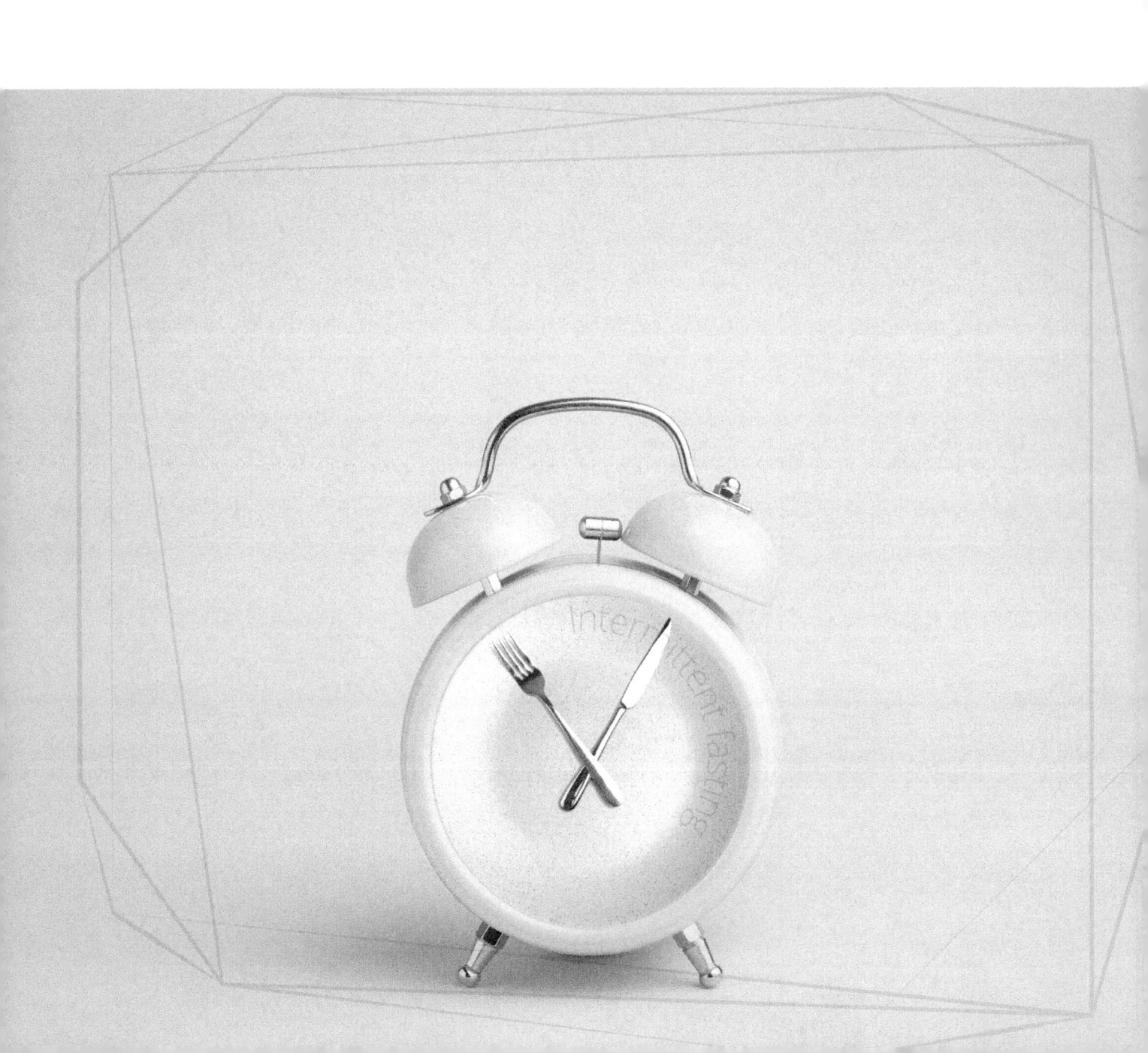

Basically, Fasting is defined as abstaining from eating anything. It is the deliberate action of depriving the body of any form of food for more than 6 hours.

Whereas Intermittent Fasting is an eating pattern that provides for a more or less long interval of fasting over a few days, alternating with a period in which you can take food without being too enslaved to the weights. This doesn't exclude that we should still take into account some precautions. Intermittent Fasting does not need to be carried out every day, but you can choose the different ways suitable for your goals and lifestyles.

In the hours of feeding, it is possible to consume almost all foods giving preference to low-calorie foods such as meat, fish, eggs, limiting simple sugars and choosing those with a low glycemic index, bread, pasta, and rice, possibly whole grains, legumes, dried and fresh fruits, good fats.

One of its forms is where the fast is carried out in a cyclic manner with the aim to reduce the overall caloric intake in a day.

The main goal is to divert the body's attention from the digestion of food. During the fasting period, in fact, a series of metabolic changes take place in the body: since there is no food left in the stomach to digest, the body focuses on the process of recovery and maintenance.

To most people, it may sound unhealthy and damaging for the body, but scientific research has proven that fasting can produce positive results on the human mind and body. According to Healthline, the American Medical-Scientific Journal, this system helps reduce overall calorie intake and, as a result, not only can help people lose weight effortlessly but can improve the overall functioning of metabolism. It can also positively affect our mind teaching self-discipline and fighting against bad eating practices and habits. It is basically an umbrella term that is used to define all voluntary forms of fasting. This dietary approach does not restrict the consumption of certain food items; rather, it works by reducing the overall food intake, leaving enough space to meet the essential nutrients the body needs. Therefore, it is proven to be far more effective and much easier in implementation, given that the dieter completely understands the nature and science of Intermittent Fasting.

Intermittent Fasting is categorized into 3 broad methods of food abstinence, including alternate-day fasting, daily restrictions, and periodic fasting. The means may vary, but the end goal of Intermittent Fasting remains the same, which is to achieve a better metabolism, healthy body weight, and active lifestyle. The American Heart Association, AHA, has also studied Intermittent Fasting and its results. According to the AHA, it can help in countering insulin resistance, cardio-metabolic diseases, and leads to weight loss. However, a question mark remains on the sustainability of this health-effective method. The 2019 research "Effects of Intermittent Fasting on health, aging, and disease" has also found Intermittent Fasting to be effective against insulin resistance, inflammation, hypertension, obesity, and dyslipidemia. However, the work on this dietary approach is still underway, and the traditional methods of fasting, which existed for almost the entire human history, in every religion from Buddhism to Jainism, Orthodox Christianity, Hinduism, and Islam, are studied to found relevance in today's age of science and technology.

## How Does It Work?

Eating is a primary need that we satisfy unceasingly from birth. Every day we introduce food into our organisms. When we eat, the metabolism activates itself to start the digestive process. This process uses a huge amount of energy. The more food we introduce, the more the body will have to work to metabolize it. If the food consumed is too much or too full of sugars and fats, the effort that the digestive system must sustain is yet greater.

When we fast, however, we stop this process and this energy dispensing. The saved energy is thus diverted to other metabolic processes, essentially of a restorative type.

Dr. Longo, Director of the Institute of Longevity at the University of Southern California, explained how, thanks to this practice, "the immune system frees itself from useless, unnecessary cells, while it is driven to put back into action naturally stem cells capable of ensuring regeneration, as was the case at the moments of birth and growth, "

The body not engaged in food digestion can better devote itself to its purification by moving toxins away through its emunctory organs. These large internal cleanings obviously have positive repercussions on the state of health of organs and tissues. The organism is detoxified and revitalized.

Intermittent Fasting is a tool that can help us activate the processes described above and face a real fast. In fact, it works between alternating periods of eating and fasting. It is a much more flexible approach, as there are many options to choose from according to body type, size, weight goals, and nutritional needs.

The human body works like a synchronized machine that requires sufficient time for self-healing and repair. When we constantly eat junk and unhealthy food or too high a quantity of food without considering our caloric needs, it leads to obesity and toxic build-up in the body. That is why fasting comes as a natural means of detoxifying the body and providing it enough time to utilize its fat deposits.

Whatever the human body consumes is ultimately broken into glucose, which is later utilized by the cells in glycolysis to release energy. As the blood glucose level rises, insulin is produced to lower the levels and allow the liver to carry out De Novo Lipogenesis (DNL), the process in which the excess glucose is turned into glycogen and ultimately stored into fat resulting in obesity. Intermittent Fasting seems to reverse this process by deliberately creating energy deprivation, which is then fulfilled by breaking down the existing fat deposits.

Intermittent Fasting works through lipolysis, the metabolic process of breaking down the fats, through enzymes and water, or hydrolysis. Fats are divided into glycerol and three fatty acids. Lipolysis takes place in our adipose tissue reserves, and it can only be initiated when the blood glucose levels drop to a sufficiently low point. That point can be achieved through fasting and exercising. When a person cuts off the external glucose supply for several hours, the body switches to lipolysis.

Fats, in fact, may be thought of as simply stored energy. When our glucose reserves run low between meals, fats are accessible and available, and it makes sense for lipolysis to occur since it will expedite the flow of these stored fats through our circulation. This "potential energy" may then be reused as fuel by breaking it down into free-moving fatty acids.

This process of breaking the fats also releases other by-products like ketones which are capable of reducing the oxidative stress of the body and help in its detoxification.

While discussing the application of this dietary approach, it is imperative to understand how Intermittent Fasting stands out from casual dieting practices. It is not mere abstinence from eating. What is eaten in this dietary lifestyle is equally important as the fasting itself. It does not result in malnutrition; rather, it promotes healthy eating along with the fast. Intermittent Fasting is divided into two different states that follow one another. The cycle starts with the "FED" state, which is followed by a "FASTING" state. The duration of the fasting state and the frequency of the fed state are established by the method of IF. The latter is characterized by high blood glucose levels, whereas during the fasting state, the body goes through a gradual decline in glucose levels. This decline in glucose signals the pancreas and the brain to meet the body's energy needs by processing the available fat molecules. However, if the fasting state is followed by a fed state in which a person binge eats food rich in carbs and fats, it will turn out to be more hazardous for their health. Therefore, the fasting period must be accompanied by a healthy diet.

## The Role of Insulin

Biologically, Intermittent Fasting works at many levels, from cellular levels to gene expression and body growth. In order to understand the science behind the workings of Intermittent Fasting, it is important to learn about the role of insulin levels, human growth hormones, cellular repair, and gene expression. Intermittent Fasting firstly lowers glucose levels, which in turn drops insulin levels. This lowering of insulin helps fat burning in the body, thus gradually curbing obesity and related disorders. Controlled levels of insulin are also responsible for preventing diabetes and insulin resistance. On the other hand, Intermittent Fasting boosts the production of Human Growth Hormones (HGH) up to 5 times. The increased production of HGH aids quick fat burning and muscle formation.

During the fasting state, the body goes into the process of self-healing at cellular levels, thus removing the unwanted, unfunctional cells and debris. This creates a cleansing effect that directly or indirectly nourishes the body and allows it to grow under reduced oxidative stress. Likewise, fasting even affects the gene expression within the human body. The cell functions according to the coding and decoding of the gene's expression; when this transcription occurs at a normal pace in a healthy environment, it automatically translates into the longevity of the cells, and fasting ensures unhindered transcription. Thus, Intermittent Fasting fights aging, cancer, and boosts the immune system by strengthening the body cells.

# CHAPTER 2

# 10 Methods to Do Intermittent Fasting

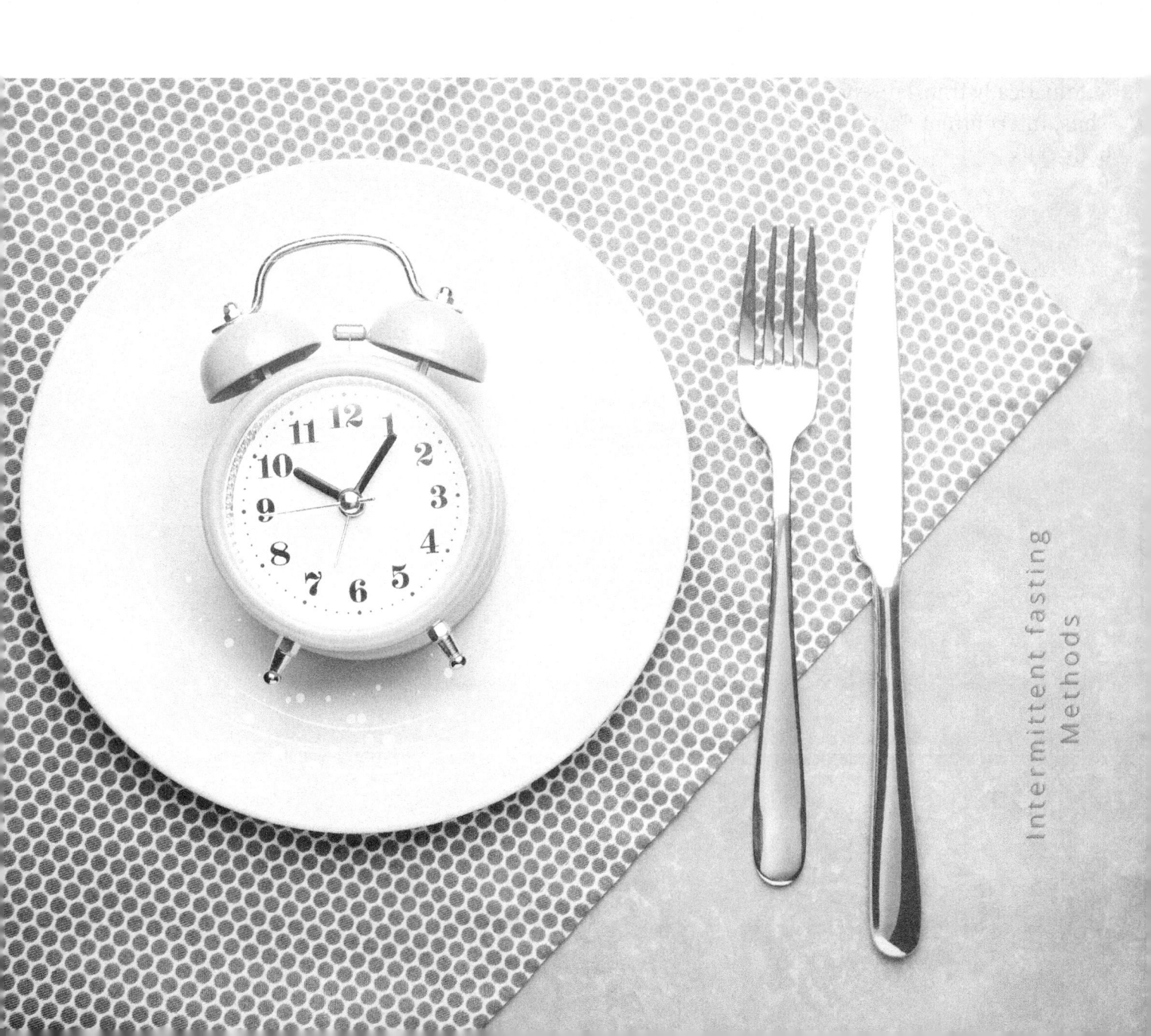

# 16:8

This method entails restricting calorie-containing foods and beverages to an eight-hour window per day and abstaining from meals for the remaining 16 hours. You may choose an 8-hour timeframe to match your daily needs. For instance, it may be between 10 a.m. and 6 p.m., or 12 a.m. and 8 p.m., and so on. Your sugar and insulin levels are lower after 16 hours of fasting, and part of your reserve glycogen has been depleted, so your body is searching for fuel. Your adipose (fat) tissue, on the other hand, has enough energy to spare. This time without meals also frees up resources for regeneration and repair by allowing your body to rest from the energy-intensive work of digestion.

## 16:8 SCHEDULE

|  | DAY 1 | DAY 2 | DAY 3 | DAY 4 | DAY 5 | DAY 6 | DAY 7 |
|---|---|---|---|---|---|---|---|
| MIDNIGHT | FAST | FAST | FAST | FAST | FAST | FAST | FAST |
| 12 AM | First Meal at 12 AM | First Meal at 12 AM | First Meal at 12 AM | First Meal at 12 AM | First Meal at 12 AM | First Meal at 12 AM | First Meal at 12 AM |
| 8 PM | Last Meal by 8 PM | Last Meal by 8 PM | Last Meal by 8 PM | Last Meal by 8 PM | Last Meal by 8 PM | Last Meal by 8 PM | Last Meal by 8 PM |
| MIDNIGHT | FAST | FAST | FAST | FAST | FAST | FAST | FAST |

### Advantages

16:8 fasting satisfies the three E's (easy to do, enjoyable, and effective). Many individuals find it simple to skip breakfast since hunger is generally lower in the morning, and the activities associated with this time of day keep their thoughts from thinking about food. Dinner may be enjoyed as a family activity. Fasting for 16 hours is also beneficial to one's health and weight reduction.

### Disadvantages

Fasting from evening until breakfast the following day demands avoiding after-dinner beverages and snacks, as well as reducing or eliminating coffee creamer. These lifestyle changes might be difficult.

# 14:10

The 10:14 diet requires you to eat all of your meals within a 10-hour window before fasting for 14 hours. For example, if your first meal is at 7:00 a.m., you must complete your last feed by 5:00 p.m. This approach is similar to the 16:8 method; however, it requires a 14-hour fast instead of 16.

"Typically, people would go for an 8 a.m. to 6 p.m. eating window," says Dr. Pam Taub, a cardiologist at the University of California, San Diego's School of Medicine and research author.

## 14:10 SCHEDULE

|  | DAY 1 | DAY 2 | DAY 3 | DAY 4 | DAY 5 | DAY 6 | DAY 7 |
|---|---|---|---|---|---|---|---|
| MIDNIGHT | FAST | FAST | FAST | FAST | FAST | FAST | FAST |
| 10 AM | First Meal at 10 AM | First Meal at 10 AM | First Meal at 10 AM | First Meal at 10 AM | First Meal at 10 AM | First Meal at 10 AM | First Meal at 10 AM |
| 8 PM | Last Meal by 8 PM | Last Meal by 8 PM | Last Meal by 8 PM | Last Meal by 8 PM | Last Meal by 8 PM | Last Meal by 8 PM | Last Meal by 8 PM |
| MIDNIGHT | FAST | FAST | FAST | FAST | FAST | FAST | FAST |

## Advantages

It's a bit simpler to follow than 16:8 since you have a larger eating window, and it very well matches how people already eat. This technique is ideal if you're new to intermittent fasting and want to test how you react when you have a specific eating schedule and can't just eat whenever the whim strikes. You can always switch to the 16:8 method later once you have tested this method.

## Disadvantages

When it comes to weight reduction, it may be less successful than the 16:8 technique, and it may be difficult for certain people to create a calorie deficit with this method.

## 12:12

The 12/12 fast is a kind of intermittent fasting in which you eat for 12 hours and fast for the remaining 12 hours of the day. It is often referred to as overnight fasting since eating is limited to a 12-hour window, and fasting occurs during the night. For example, if you complete your supper at 8 p.m., you can have your breakfast at 8 a.m. the next day.

This is an excellent place to start if you are new to fasting. Consider it an overnight fast, similar to what you would do before a blood test. If your doctor has scheduled a blood test for the following morning, he or she may instruct you to quit eating after supper and not eat again until the morning of the test. It does not get much easier than that to keep a 12-hour fast.

### 12:12 SCHEDULE

|  | DAY 1 | DAY 2 | DAY 3 | DAY 4 | DAY 5 | DAY 6 | DAY 7 |
|---|---|---|---|---|---|---|---|
| MIDNIGHT | FAST | FAST | FAST | FAST | FAST | FAST | FAST |
| 8 AM | First Meal at 8 AM | First Meal at 8 AM | First Meal at 8 AM | First Meal at 8 AM | First Meal at 8 AM | First Meal at 8 AM | First Meal at 8 AM |
| 8 PM | Last Meal by 8 PM | Last Meal by 8 PM | Last Meal by 8 PM | Last Meal by 8 PM | Last Meal by 8 PM | Last Meal by 8 PM | Last Meal by 8 PM |
| MIDNIGHT | FAST | FAST | FAST | FAST | FAST | FAST | FAST |

### Advantages

You may eat 3 or even more meals as you usually would throughout the day as long as you limit your calorie consumption to a 12-hour timeframe.

### Disadvantages

While this relatively brief time without eating may assist in balancing sugar levels and maintaining weight, the overall weight reduction and health advantages of IF will not be fulfilled by this approach.

# The 5:2 Diet

The 5:2 diet, also known as the Fast Diet, is based on the principle of fasting for 2 days a week and eating properly for the other 5 days. Dr. Michael Mosley developed this variation on alternate-day fasting.

Dr. Mosley is a British television personality and former medical doctor who published "The Fast Diet," a best-selling book. The 5:2 diet strategy outlined in the book allows you to normally eat for five days and limit your calories intake for two days, which is 500 for women (600 for men). According to Dr. Mosley's strategy, eating "normally" implies ingesting the number of calories your body requires to accomplish everyday tasks. That implies you shouldn't eat too much on non-fasting days. Instead, you are urged to eat a variety of meals in sensible quantities.

## 5:2 SCHEDULE

| DAY 1 | DAY 2 | DAY 3 | DAY 4 | DAY 5 | DAY 6 | DAY 7 |
|---|---|---|---|---|---|---|
| EAT NORMALLY | FAST or Eat max. 500 calories (men 600 calories) | EAT NORMALLY | EAT NORMALLY | FAST or Eat max. 500 calories (men 600 calories) | EAT NORMALLY | EAT NORMALLY |

## Advantages

Unlike other kinds of alternate day fasting, the 5:2 approach restricts calories just on 2 days of the week rather than every other day. Even though the effort is still necessary, this approach is the least restrictive and hence the most accessible for people interested in alternate-day fasting.

## Disadvantages

You may have adverse effects such as irritation, hunger, or problems sleeping, as with any high-calorie restriction. Furthermore, for some individuals, 5 days of "regular" eating might be a steep slope in relation to food decisions. It is natural to want to treat oneself after a hard day's work, which may translate into consuming more unhealthy food than usual on non-fasting days.

# The Warrior Diet (20:4)

Ori Hofmekler, a fitness specialist, developed the Warrior Diet in the early 2000s, based on his own experiences with the diet, which are detailed in his book of the same name. The diet consisted of 20 hours of "underfeeding" meals of dairy, eggs, fruits, and vegetables and a four-hour "overfeeding" window. This diet is inspired by ancient warrior tribes that ate little portions of full, unprocessed meals throughout the day and one huge meal in the evening.

The classic Warrior Diet recommended a specific eating plan that included a big, drawn-out evening meal rich in protein, unrefined carbs, and healthy fats. Many individuals nowadays have adapted this diet, taking it to extremes, fasting for 20 consecutive hours. They consider it as a technique to drive their bodies to a greater degree of fat burning and cellular regeneration, despite the fact that little research has been conducted to back up these claims.

## WARRIOR DIET SCHEDULE

|  | DAY 1 | DAY 2 | DAY 3 | DAY 4 | DAY 5 | DAY 6 | DAY 7 |
|---|---|---|---|---|---|---|---|
| MIDNIGHT | FAST | FAST | FAST | FAST | FAST | FAST | FAST |
|  | or | or | or | or | or | or | or |
|  | Eat small amounts of dairy, raw fruits or vegetables | Eat small amounts of dairy, raw fruits or vegetables | Eat small amounts of dairy, raw fruits or vegetables | Eat small amounts of dairy, raw fruits or vegetables | Eat small amounts of dairy, raw fruits or vegetables | Eat small amounts of dairy, raw fruits or vegetables | Eat small amounts of dairy, raw fruits or vegetables |
| 16 PM – 20 PM | Large Meal | Large Meal | Large Meal | Large Meal | Large Meal | Large Meal | Large Meal |
| MIDNIGHT | FAST | FAST | FAST | FAST | FAST | FAST | FAST |

## Advantages

Those with a slow metabolism may notice that fasting for 20 hours is all their body needs to lose weight. It might also be claimed that the extra hours of low blood glucose and insulin levels might help those with diabetes.

## Disadvantages

If you start this strategy too soon, you may develop hunger and cravings, which may result in binge eating. If you view a 20:4 fast as an advanced skill level to practice once you have been comfortable with 16:8 fasting, you will have the best results.

# One Meal a Day (OMAD)

The abbreviation OMAD refers to "one meal a day." Because that meal is usually eaten in an hour, OMAD may also be regarded as a 23-hour fast or 23:1 fasting. This is the most stringent kind of time-restricted eating method.

## ONE MEAL A DAY SCHEDULE

|  | DAY 1 | DAY 2 | DAY 3 | DAY 4 | DAY 5 | DAY 6 | DAY 7 |
|---|---|---|---|---|---|---|---|
| MIDNIGHT | FAST | FAST | FAST | FAST | FAST | FAST | FAST |
| 20 PM | Large Meal | Large Meal | Large Meal | Large Meal | Large Meal | Large Meal | Large Meal |
| MIDNIGHT | FAST | FAST | FAST | FAST | FAST | FAST | FAST |

## Advantages

Including an OMAD fast in your weekly schedule may assist you in breaking through a weight-loss plateau. If you are traveling or have a very hectic day ahead of you, OMAD makes life easier by minimizing the time spent preparing and consuming meals.

## Disadvantages

When you limit your calorie intake to 1 hour per day, it is difficult to receive most of the vitamins and calories you need to keep your metabolism from slowing down. If you use this strategy on a regular basis, you will get the best results if you keep track of your body fat % to ensure that you are shedding fat rather than muscle.

# Fasting Mimicking Diet

Dr. Valter Longo, an Italian scientist, and researcher developed the Fasting Mimicking Diet. He wanted to recreate the advantages of fasting while also supplying nourishment to the body. His changes eliminate the calorie shortage that comes with other kinds of fasting.

The Fasting Mimicking regimen is based on extensive research and clinical investigations. Dr. Longo promotes the ProLon Fasting Mimicking Diet, a 5-day weight reduction regimen based on the concepts of fast mimicking, via L-Nutra, a nutrition technology firm he founded.

ProLon's Fasting Mimicking Diet plan contains prepared low-calorie meal kits for five days. All meals and snacks are made with healthy foods and are plant-based. The meal kits are low in carbohydrates and protein but rich in healthy fats such as olive oil and flaxseed.

Dieters eat just the contents of the meal kit throughout the five-day period.

After glycogen reserves are exhausted, your body will produce energy from noncarbohydrate sources due to the meals' low calorie, high fat, low carbohydrate composition. This is known as gluconeogenesis.

This calorie restriction replicates the physiological reaction of the body to conventional fasting techniques, such as cell regeneration, reduced inflammation, and fat reduction.

The ProLon five-day detox is not a one-time event; it must be repeated every one to six months to get the best benefits.

Below you can find the official web page of the diet

https://prolonfast.com/

## Advantages

ProLon users have experienced increased energy, mental alertness, and focus, in addition to weight loss. Fewer food cravings and improved eating habits, the capacity to be more conscious during meals, greater drive to embrace a healthy lifestyle, a clearer understanding of food proportioning, and a greater capacity to resist sugar foods are all stated advantages participants have experienced after leaving the program.

## Disadvantages

You may suffer side effects such as a minor headache, tiredness, and trouble focusing when using ProLon. In addition, unlike other diets that focus on lifestyle improvements, ProLon is only intended to be utilized for a limited time. ProLon is not the diet plan for you if you are seeking something you can stick to long-term.

# Eat Stop Eat (24 hours)

Eat Stop Eat is a novel method of Intermittent Fasting in which a maximum of 2 non-consecutive complete fasting days is included each week. For example, you could eat regularly until 7 p.m. on Saturday, then fast until 7 p.m. on Sunday before returning to regular eating. This would be one of the two fasting days.

Brad Pilon, writer of the famous and appropriately named book "Eat Stop Eat," created it. The Eat Stop Eat technique is not your usual weight-reduction plan, according to Pilon. Instead, it is an opportunity to reconsider what you have been taught about mealtime and frequency, as well as how it connects to your health.

Pilon also give some flexibility; If you can't make it for the whole 24 hours, he believes that anything between 20 and 24 hours would work.

## EAT-STOP-EAT SCHEDULE

| DAY 1 | DAY 2 | DAY 3 | DAY 4 | DAY 5 | DAY 6 | DAY 7 |
|---|---|---|---|---|---|---|
| EAT NORMALLY | 24-HOUR FAST | EAT NORMALLY | EAT NORMALLY | 24-HOUR FAST | EAT NORMALLY | EAT NORMALLY |

### Advantages

It is easier to adopt, and there is no need to track calories. This is the best benefit. It's less complicated than diets that require you to restrict an entire food category, such as fat or carbohydrates.

### Disadvantages

Fasting for 24-hour intervals each week may affect family dinners and social contact with friends, which can greatly affect your mood

The transition to this diet possibly has side effects such as dehydration, hunger, and vitamin shortages. According to experts, this is related to your body's need for time to adjust to utilizing ketones as an energy source rather than glucose.

## Alternate-Day Fasting

Alternate-day fasting (ADF) is done by switching between fasting and non-fasting days, as the name implies. Every other day you must entirely refrain from caloric food and drink, while the days between them, you can eat as you typically would.

You are free to modify these guidelines as you see fit, just like you would with any other fasting regimen. Especially at the beginning, it may be difficult for you to spend a whole day without eating (say "Hi" to your growling stomach). So, on fasting days, you should attempt to eat but restrict your calories.

### ALTERNATE-DAY FASTING SCHEDULE

| DAY 1 | DAY 2 | DAY 3 | DAY 4 | DAY 5 | DAY 6 | DAY 7 |
|---|---|---|---|---|---|---|
| EAT NORMALLY | 24-Hour Fast *or* Eat only a few hundred calories | EAT NORMALLY | EAT NORMALLY | 24-Hour Fast *or* Eat only a few hundred calories | EAT NORMALLY | EAT NORMALLY |

### Advantages

Alternate-day fasting is the most researched fasting strategy, demonstrating good health and weight-loss effects. Many individuals find that an alternate-day fasting habit is easier to keep than more standard diets that limit calories every day.

### Disadvantages

It is likely that going without meals for more than a day will result in muscle mass loss. You need self-control, and hunger may arise on fasting days. Please keep in mind that the studies on this and other kinds of alternate-day fasting were conducted over a period of several months, so commitment may be required to reap the full advantages.

# Meal Skipping

Meal skipping is an incredibly adaptable kind of fasting that offers all Intermittent Fasting advantages but with fewer restrictions. If you do not have a regular schedule or do not think a tighter version of the IF Diet would work for you, meal skipping from time to time is an option.

Meal skipping is a terrific approach for many individuals to respond to their bodies and follow their natural impulses. They just do not eat that meal if they are not hungry.

Skipping one or two meals whenever you feel ok with that is essentially a spontaneous intermittent fast. This may result more natural than the other fasting techniques.

## MEAL SKIPPING SCHEDULE

| DAY 1 | DAY 2 | DAY 3 | DAY 4 | DAY 5 | DAY 6 | DAY 7 |
|---|---|---|---|---|---|---|
| Breakfast | Meal Skipped | Breakfast | Breakfast | Breakfast | Breakfast | Breakfast |
| Lunch | Lunch | Lunch | Lunch | Lunch | Lunch | Meal Skipped |
| Dinner | Dinner | Dinner | Meal Skipped | Dinner | Dinner | Dinner |

### Advantages

This is a very flexible method of intermittent fasting and could be helpful for beginners. You can choose which meals to miss based on your hunger level or time constraints.

### Disadvantages

Skipping meals may cause blood sugar fluctuations, which can lead to bingeing and overeating later in the day. Breakfast skippers have been shown to snack more and make unhealthy choices between meals.

# CHAPTER 3

# Food to Eat and Avoid on Intermittent Fasting

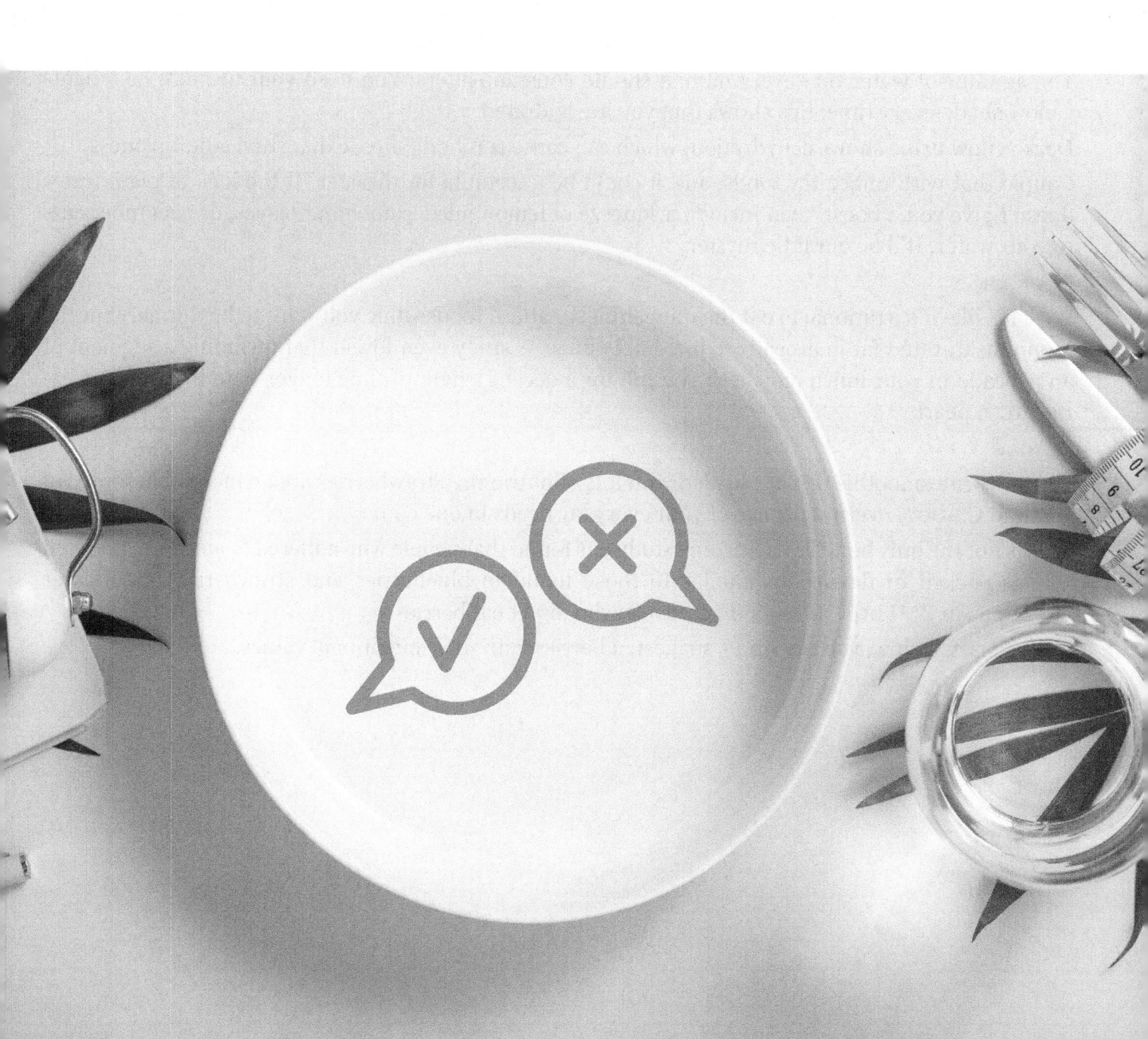

# What to Eat

Intermittent fasting is an eating pattern, not a diet. You may be unaware of what to consume during an intermittent fast because the techniques instruct you on when to eat but not on what foods to include in your diet.

Without defined dietary restrictions, it's possible to have the idea that one may eat anything they want. Others may have difficulty selecting the "appropriate" meals and beverages as a result of this.

These not only damage your weight-loss attempts, but they also increase your chances of being undernourished or overnourished.

Eating during intermittent fasting is about being healthy rather than reducing weight quickly. As a result, it is essential to select nutrient-dense meals such as vegetables, fruits, lean meats, and healthy fats.

On the following pages, you can find a list of foods that are perfect for your nutrition while you are following one of the intermittent fasting methods:

### Water

Despite the reality that you aren't eating, it's imperative to keep yourself hydrated with water for many reasons, such as for the vitality of every important organ in your body.

The amount of water that every human should consume alters. You need your urine to be a light-yellow shade every time; this shows that you are hydrated.

Dark yellow urine shows dehydration, which can cause cerebral pains, exhaustion, and tipsiness.

Couple that with unhealthy foods, and it could be a formula for disaster. If the idea of plain water doesn't give you a boost, then include a squeeze of lemon juice, some mint leaves, or cucumber cuts to your water. It'll be our little mystery.

### Avocado

It seems like it's irrational to eat the unhealthiest natural foods while you want to be thinner, but the monounsaturated fat in avocado is incredibly huge. A study even found that including a segment of an avocado in your lunch may keep you full for a decent length of time longer than if you didn't eat the green pearl.

### Berries

Your favorite smoothie drink is loaded with lots of nutrients. Strawberries are an incredible source of Vitamin C, 100% overindulgence of your everyday needs in one cup.

This is not the only benefit; an ongoing study has found that people who adhered to an eating regimen that is packed in flavonoids, similar to those found in blueberries and strawberries, had lesser elevations in BMI over 14 years than people who didn't eat berries.

In the charts below, you can find 5 suggested berries with their nutritional values.

| Strawberries (1 cup) | Raspberries (1 cup) | Blackberries (1 cup) | Blueberries (1 cup) | Goji Berries (1 cup) |
|---|---|---|---|---|
| • Calories 49 | • Calories 64 | • Calories 62 | • Calories 83 | • Calories 100 |
| • Fat 0,46g | • Fat 0,8g | • Fat 0,71g | • Fat 0,48g | • Fat 0g |
| • Carbs 11,67g | • Carbs 14,69g | • Carbs 13,84g | • Carbs 21,01g | • Carbs 22g |
| • Protein 1,02g | • Protein 1,48g | • Protein 2g | • Protein 1,07g | • Protein 4g |

## Leafy Veggies

Veggies like broccoli, Brussels sprouts, and cauliflower are, for the most part, packed with fiber. At the point when you're eating inconsistently, it's vital to eat fiber-rich foods that will keep you normal and avoid blockage.

It can also make you feel full, which is something you may need in case you can't eat again for 16 hours. In the charts below, you can find the 10 suggested leafy veggies with their nutritional values.

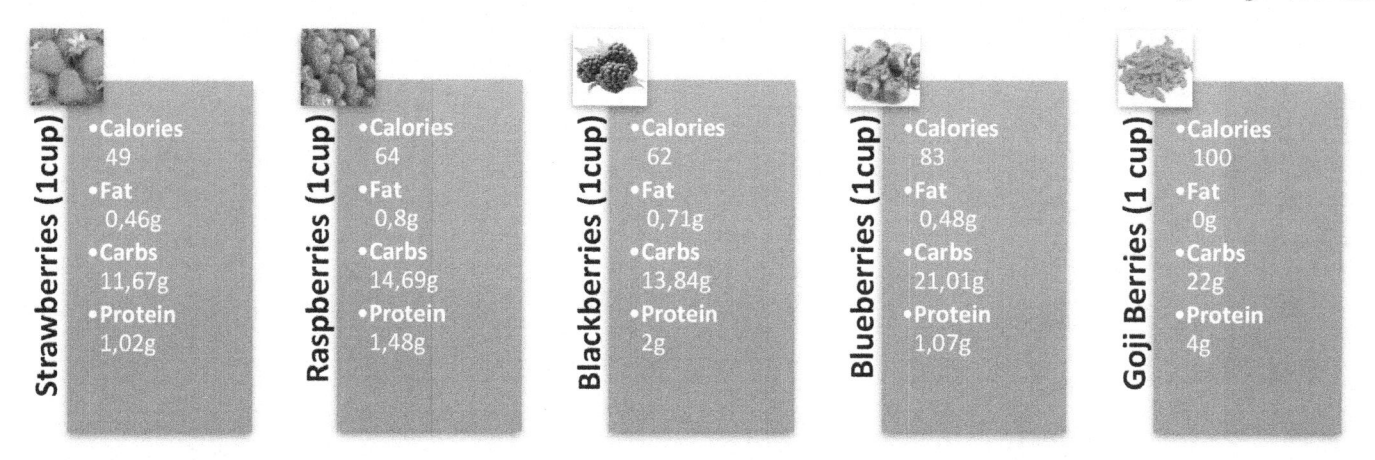

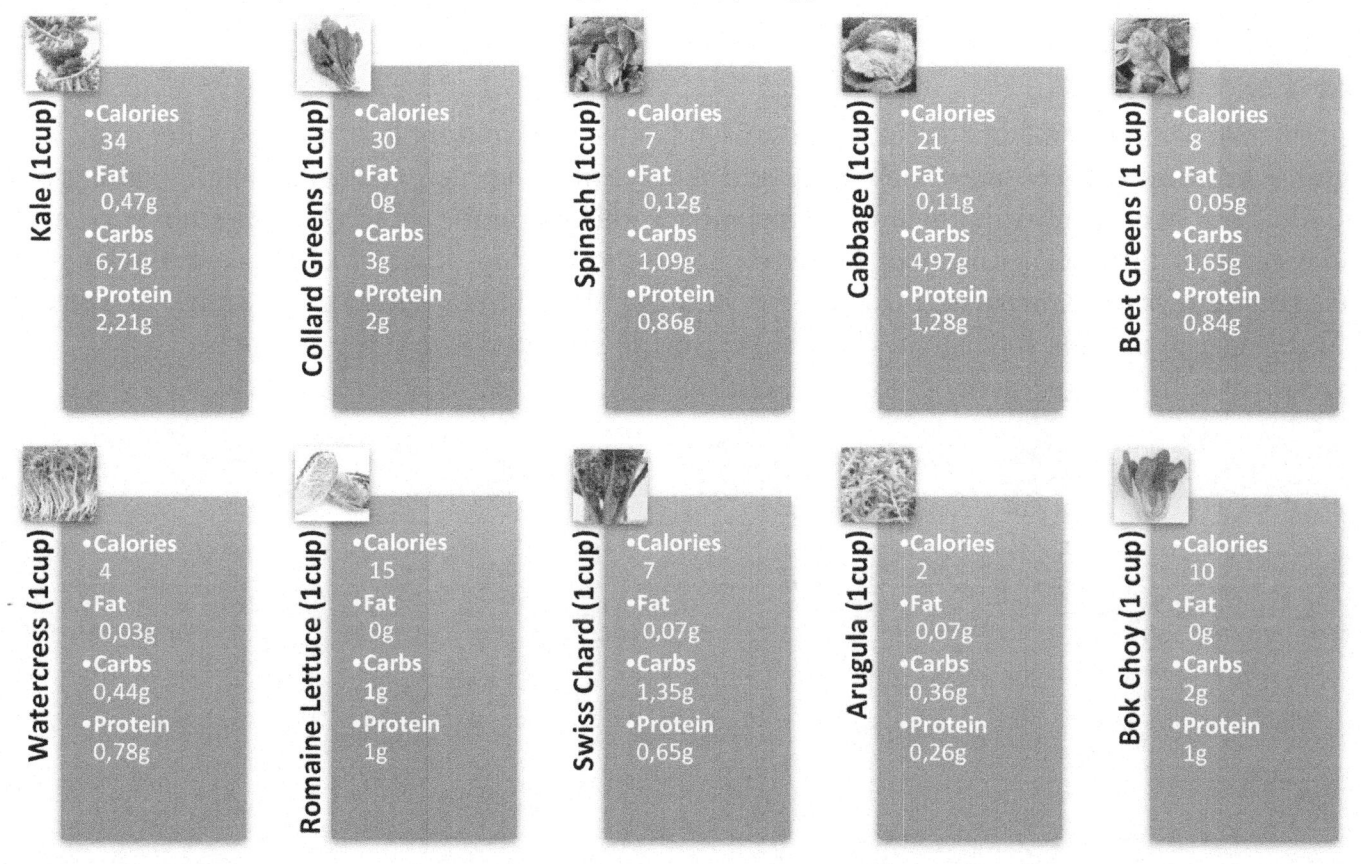

| Kale (1cup) | Collard Greens (1cup) | Spinach (1cup) | Cabbage (1cup) | Beet Greens (1 cup) |
|---|---|---|---|---|
| • Calories 34 | • Calories 30 | • Calories 7 | • Calories 21 | • Calories 8 |
| • Fat 0,47g | • Fat 0g | • Fat 0,12g | • Fat 0,11g | • Fat 0,05g |
| • Carbs 6,71g | • Carbs 3g | • Carbs 1,09g | • Carbs 4,97g | • Carbs 1,65g |
| • Protein 2,21g | • Protein 2g | • Protein 0,86g | • Protein 1,28g | • Protein 0,84g |

| Watercress (1cup) | Romaine Lettuce (1cup) | Swiss Chard (1cup) | Arugula (1cup) | Bok Choy (1 cup) |
|---|---|---|---|---|
| • Calories 4 | • Calories 15 | • Calories 7 | • Calories 2 | • Calories 10 |
| • Fat 0,03g | • Fat 0g | • Fat 0,07g | • Fat 0,07g | • Fat 0g |
| • Carbs 0,44g | • Carbs 1g | • Carbs 1,35g | • Carbs 0,36g | • Carbs 2g |
| • Protein 0,78g | • Protein 1g | • Protein 0,65g | • Protein 0,26g | • Protein 1g |

## Whole Grains

Being on an eating plan and eating carbohydrates are 2 concepts that seem to have a place in 2 separate basins, however not generally! Whole grains are wealthy in fiber and protein, so eating a little goes far in keeping you full. Additionally, another study recommends that eating whole grains rather than refined grains may fire up your digestion. In the charts below, you can find 10 suggested whole grains with their nutritional values when they are cooked.

**Bulgur (1cup)**
- Calories 151
- Fat 0,44g
- Carbs 33,82g
- Protein 5,61g

**Pearl Barley (1cup)**
- Calories 193
- Fat 0,69g
- Carbs 44,31g
- Protein 3,55g

**Quinoa (1cup)**
- Calories 229
- Fat 3,55g
- Carbs 42,17g
- Protein 8,01g

**Buckwheat (1cup)**
- Calories 155
- Fat 1,04g
- Carbs 33,5g
- Protein 5,68g

**Oatmeal (1 cup)**
- Calories 145
- Fat 2,39g
- Carbs 25,37g
- Protein 6,06g

**Brown Rice (1cup)**
- Calories 216
- Fat 1,76g
- Carbs 44,77g
- Protein 5,03g

**Wild Rice (1cup)**
- Calories 166
- Fat 0,56g
- Carbs 35g
- Protein 6,54g

**Corn (1cup)**
- Calories 132
- Fat 1,82g
- Carbs 29,29g
- Protein 4,96g

**Couscous (1cup)**
- Calories 176
- Fat 0,25g
- Carbs 36,46g
- Protein 5,95g

**Farro (1 cup)**
- Calories 200
- Fat 1g
- Carbs 44g
- Protein 5g

## Beans and Legumes

Your likable bean stew might be your greatest friend in the Intermittent Fasting way of life. Beans and legumes are good sources of carbohydrates and supply energy for action. While I am not telling you to carbo-load, it certainly wouldn't hurt to include several low-calorie carbohydrates, similar to beans and vegetables, into your eating plan. Moreover, foods such as chickpeas, dark beans, peas, and lentils have been shown to diminish excess fats, even without calorie limitation. In the chart below, you can find 10 suggested beans and legumes with their nutritional values when they are cooked.

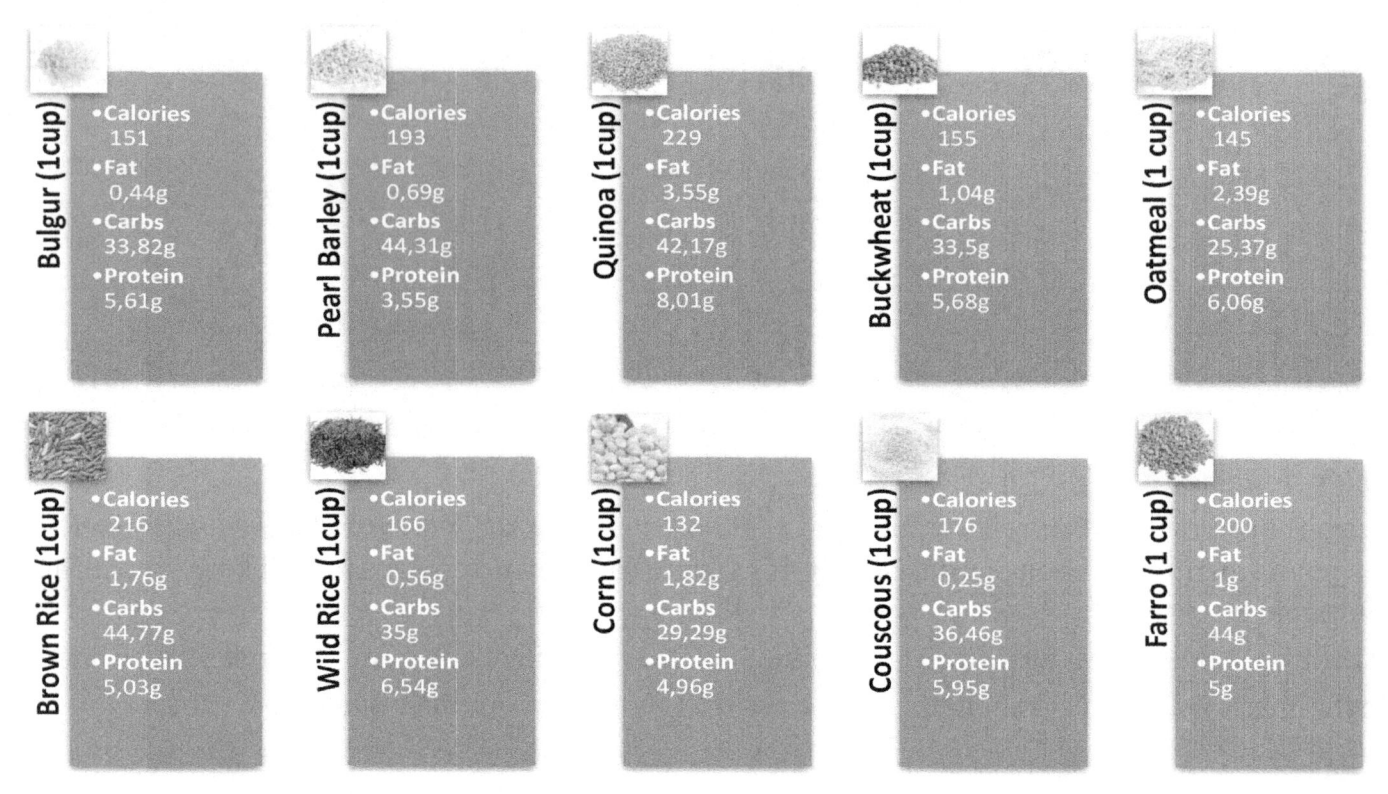

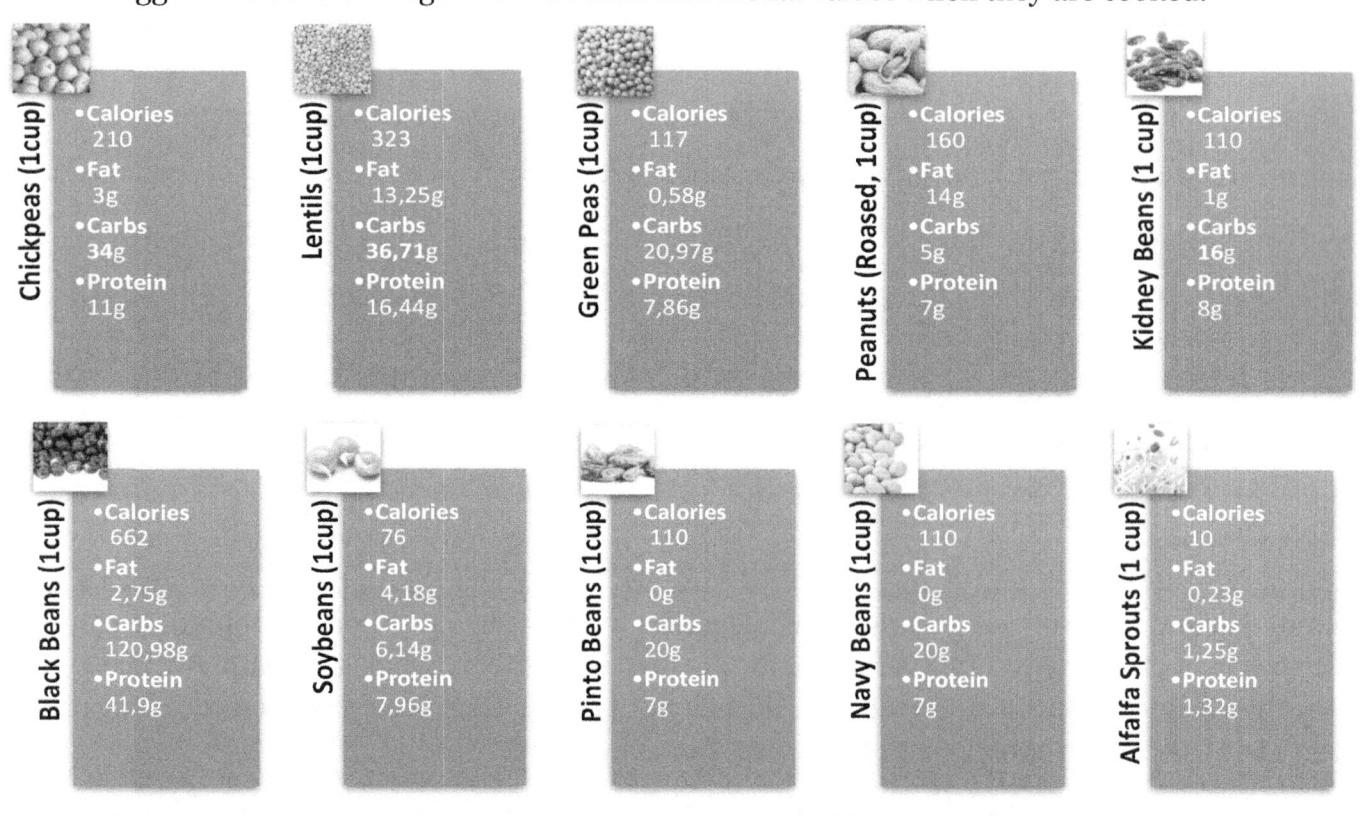

**Chickpeas (1cup)**
- Calories 210
- Fat 3g
- Carbs 34g
- Protein 11g

**Lentils (1cup)**
- Calories 323
- Fat 13,25g
- Carbs 36,71g
- Protein 16,44g

**Green Peas (1cup)**
- Calories 117
- Fat 0,58g
- Carbs 20,97g
- Protein 7,86g

**Peanuts (Roasted, 1cup)**
- Calories 160
- Fat 14g
- Carbs 5g
- Protein 7g

**Kidney Beans (1 cup)**
- Calories 110
- Fat 1g
- Carbs 16g
- Protein 8g

**Black Beans (1cup)**
- Calories 662
- Fat 2,75g
- Carbs 120,98g
- Protein 41,9g

**Soybeans (1cup)**
- Calories 76
- Fat 4,18g
- Carbs 6,14g
- Protein 7,96g

**Pinto Beans (1cup)**
- Calories 110
- Fat 0g
- Carbs 20g
- Protein 7g

**Navy Beans (1cup)**
- Calories 110
- Fat 0g
- Carbs 20g
- Protein 7g

**Alfalfa Sprouts (1 cup)**
- Calories 10
- Fat 0,23g
- Carbs 1,25g
- Protein 1,32g

## Fish

Every person should consume eight ounces of fish every week. In addition to the fact that it is rich in fats and protein, it also has measures of vitamin D. What's more, if there is a chance, you're eating a limited amount of food throughout the day, and you can consume some food supplements; however, are you getting good value for your money? Also, constraining your calorie intake may upset your stomach or mind, and fish is frequently viewed as a "brain food."

## Eggs

A huge egg has 6 grams of protein and cooks in minutes. Getting as much protein as could sensibly be expected is noteworthy for keeping full and building muscle. One study found that men who had an egg for breakfast rather than a bagel were less hungry and ate less to the extent of the day. At the end of the day, when you're probing for something to do during your fasting period, why not hard-boil an egg?

## Nuts

They may be higher in calories than numerous other snacks; however, nuts contain something that most inferior food doesn't contain. Research suggests that polyunsaturated fat in nuts can change the physiological markers for yearning and satiety.

What's more, let's say you're stressed over calories, don't be! A recent report found that a one-ounce serving of almonds has 20% fewer calories than recorded on it. Essentially, the moment you bite, it doesn't wholly take apart the almond cell dividers, leaving a segment of the nut unblemished and unabsorbed during processing.

In the chart below, you can find 10 suggested Nuts with their nutritional values.

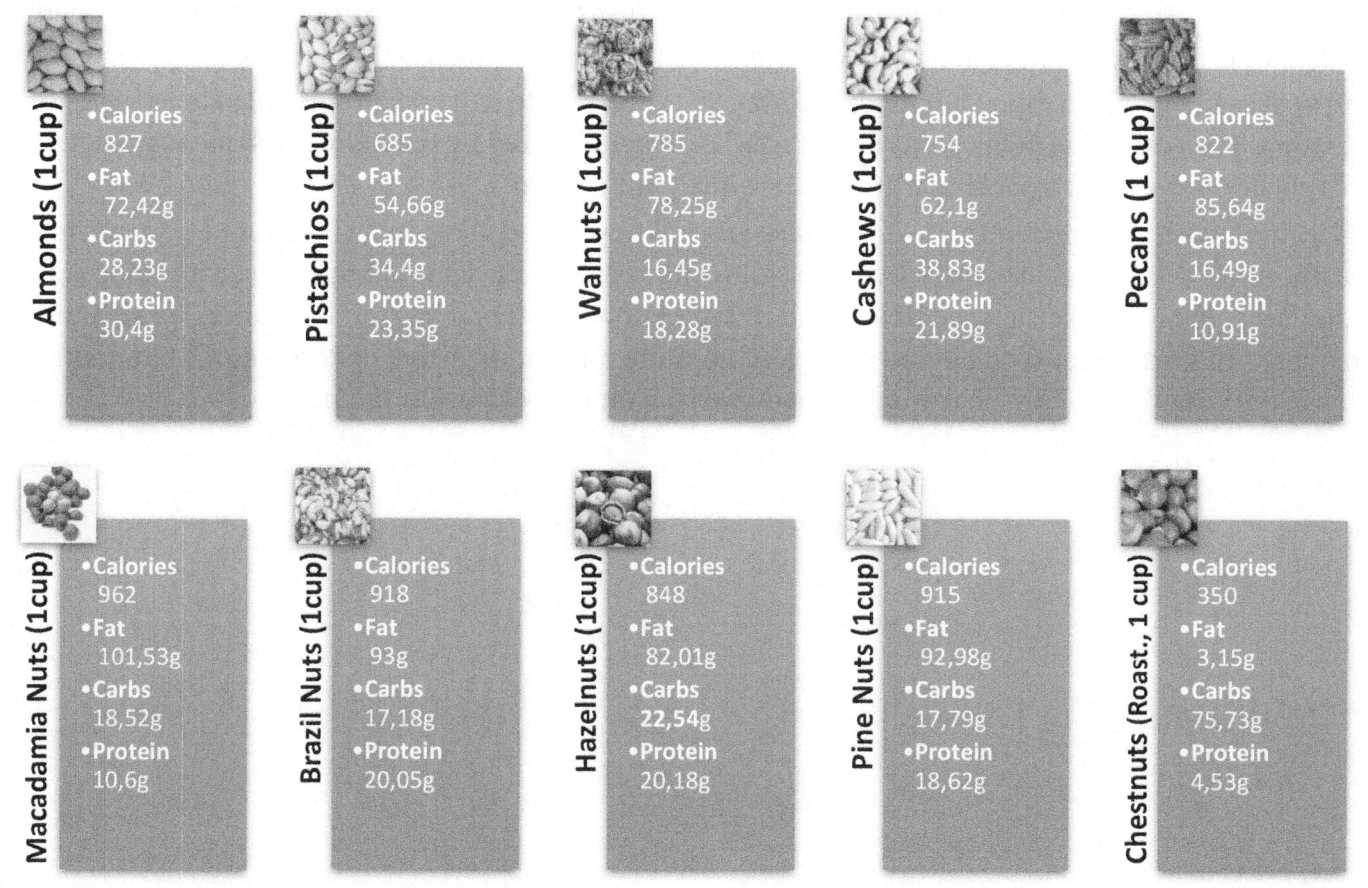

**Almonds (1 cup)**
- Calories 827
- Fat 72,42g
- Carbs 28,23g
- Protein 30,4g

**Pistachios (1 cup)**
- Calories 685
- Fat 54,66g
- Carbs 34,4g
- Protein 23,35g

**Walnuts (1 cup)**
- Calories 785
- Fat 78,25g
- Carbs 16,45g
- Protein 18,28g

**Cashews (1 cup)**
- Calories 754
- Fat 62,1g
- Carbs 38,83g
- Protein 21,89g

**Pecans (1 cup)**
- Calories 822
- Fat 85,64g
- Carbs 16,49g
- Protein 10,91g

**Macadamia Nuts (1 cup)**
- Calories 962
- Fat 101,53g
- Carbs 18,52g
- Protein 10,6g

**Brazil Nuts (1 cup)**
- Calories 918
- Fat 93g
- Carbs 17,18g
- Protein 20,05g

**Hazelnuts (1 cup)**
- Calories 848
- Fat 82,01g
- Carbs 22,54g
- Protein 20,18g

**Pine Nuts (1 cup)**
- Calories 915
- Fat 92,98g
- Carbs 17,79g
- Protein 18,62g

**Chestnuts (Roast., 1 cup)**
- Calories 350
- Fat 3,15g
- Carbs 75,73g
- Protein 4,53g

# Foods to Avoid

You often hear health experts demonizing sugar and carbohydrates. Now, it should be said that sugar and carbohydrates are not necessarily bad. They become a problem when they are consumed in excess. When you eat too many of these foods, your body has to play catch up. Naturally, this is where you accumulate fat, gain weight, and see the adverse effects of an unhealthy diet. So, the Intermittent Fasting approach calls for you to avoid, or at least significantly reduce, the following foods:

**Foods Loaded with Carbohydrates**

White bread, or anything baked, is usually loaded with a high amount of carbohydrates,

**White Starchy Foods**

This includes past and potatoes. Starch is metabolized as glucose and immediately goes into fat stores.

**Salty Foods**

There's nothing wrong with salt unless you eat too much of it. Salting foods to taste is fine. However, excessively salty foods are not only addictive, but they affect your blood pressure and heart health. To cook would be better to switch to one of the low-sodium salts.

**Greasy Foods**

Deep-fried and very greasy foods, while tasty, are high in unhealthy fats. These types of fats lead to high cholesterol.

These foods are enemy number one for blood vessel health. They generally lead to poor circulation.

**Sugary Drinks and Alcohol**

By "sugary," we mean things like sodas and iced teas. These are loaded with sugar and other chemicals. Also, alcoholic beverages end up accumulating fat in a heartbeat. Now, consuming moderate amounts of alcohol is fine unless you have particular diseases that prohibit its use. In fact, a glass of wine (☺) per week will not affect your diet much. However, excessive alcohol consumption leads to increased fat gains. The reasoning behind this is that alcohol is metabolized by the body the same way sugar is. So, this implies you'll be packing extra glucose into your system.

Also, check with your doctor to see if you have any unknown food allergies. Unfortunately, many folks out there go through their entire lives not knowing they are, in fact, allergic to certain foods. For instance, some folks are lactose intolerant but don't know it. Other common food allergies are gluten and corn. In particular, corn allergies can lead to quite a bit of digestive distress and inflammation. This is important to note as many of the foods we consume have corn in them.

# CHAPTER 4

# Benefits of Intermittent Fasting

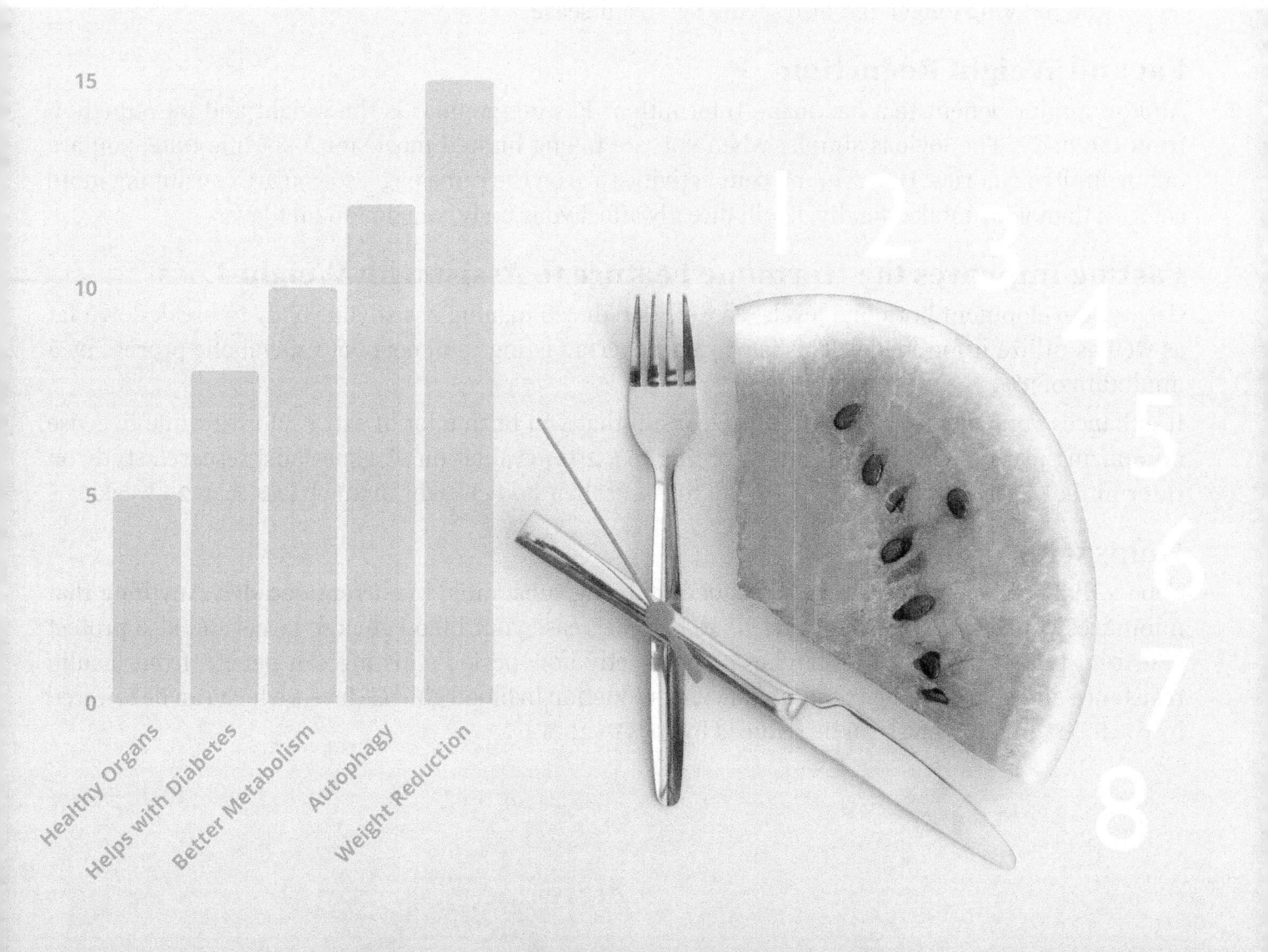

There are excellent bargains of various diet plans that you can pick from. Some help you limit your carb intake and focus on good fats and healthy proteins. Some will restrict your fat consumption and also concentrate on healthy and balanced superb carbs.

With all the alternatives in the industry, and with at least a few of them being reputable selections for lowering weight, you might ask yourself why you must choose Intermittent Fasting. Let's have a look at the various benefits of periodic fasting and also how it will make a distinction in your health.

## Change the Feature of Cells, Hormones, and Genetics

Numerous things take place in your body when you do not consume food for some time. Your body will start initiating procedures for cell repair work as well as altering some of your hormonal agent degrees, which makes maintaining body fat much easier to obtain accessibility to.

Other adjustments that can occur in the body contain:

- **Insulin degrees:** your insulin degrees will come by a reasonable bit, which makes it easier for the body to melt fat.
- **Human development hormone agent:** the blood levels of the hormonal development agent can significantly rise. Greater levels of this hormonal representative can assist in building muscular tissue as well as burn fat.
- **Mobile repair work:** the body will certainly begin important mobile repair procedures, such as getting rid of all the waste from cells.
- **Gene expression:** some helpful modifications happen in countless genetics that will assist you in living longer and also secure against disease.

## Fat and Weight Reduction

Another major benefit that has made Intermittent Fasting popular is the weight and fat reduction from the body. The logic is simple: when you are taking limited meals for a specific time, you are taking limited calories. However, all your activities are on the same page, so you are consuming more calories than your intake; finally, it will directly affect your body, weight, and fat layers.

## Fasting Improves the Hormone Feature to Assist with Weight-Loss

Greater development hormone levels, as well as reduced insulin, assist your body to break down fat as well as utilize it for energy. This is why short-term fasting can boost your metabolic process by a minimum of 3%.

It enhances your metabolic rate to make certain that you burn a lot of extra calories while likewise minimizing just how much you eat. According to a 2014 evaluation of a specialist research study on Intermittent Fasting, people could lose up to 8% of their body weight in much less than 24 weeks.

## Helps with Diabetes

Type-2 diabetes is an illness that has ended up being substantial in current decades. Anything that minimizes your insulin resistance needs to help decrease your blood glucose levels and also protect you from type 2 diabetes. Researches show exactly how periodic fasting can benefit from insulin resistance and also can help create an amazing reduction in blood glucose levels which can be lowered by 6% to 3%. Insulin level can be reduced by 31% to 20%.

## Purification of the Body

This process helps you to purify the body and organs as well. When we make a meal for the first 8 hours, and then we fast for the next 16 hours in a day, it means that we will take selective food only. The food should be something that takes time to digest and provides us the energy, gradually. Moreover, during the fasting timings, we will focus on detox water, herbal tea, or other electrolytes to maintain the glucose level. The selection of food will definitely exclude fast food and energy drinks from the diet. In the end, we will be relying on natural options like fruits, whole wheat, and vegetables; it will help to boost metabolism and reduce the overall toxins.

## Inner Cleansing

For a healthy and presentable personality, we mainly focus on the outer cleansing that starts from the apparel to the skin. However, to sustain your personality, you should have inner cleansing that purifies your organs and keeps your blood clean as well. Intermittent Fasting plays an integral role in cleansing your body from inside that impacts every cell and its formation too. From the blood cells to the tissues and even organs, it makes everything clean and purified in your body.

However, this purification is directly linked with your routine and the food intake you are having in the period. Make sure that you are not going to compromise the routine, and you are following the best diet plan for Intermittent Fasting. It will make you get the desired results in the end.

## Healthy Organs

Due to our poor diet management and lifestyle, we commonly face a number of health issues and problems such as kidney stones, liver issues, diabetes, heart problems, hypertension, and so on. All these issues are related to the poor performing organs in our bodies.

These organs are mostly under threat due to careless diet plans and poor weight management as well. With the support of Intermittent Fasting, we can make our organs healthy and take care of the essentials that keep up running in our life. Studies evaluate that people following a healthy diet with Intermittent Fasting have organs with better health and do not face many health-related issues. In fact, it helps them to recover from any damage that happens to the organs by keeping things in control and schedule.

## Better Immune System

Most of the problems that come up to our body are due to a weak immune system; it increases the chances of infections and bacterial attacks. Intermittent Fasting is not just limited to weight control or organ purification. In fact, it is linked with the overall immune system and body balance.

## Better Metabolism

When you are not overloading your stomach with a lot of food and giving it time to work properly and digest it, then you are working to improve your metabolism. Eventually, the stomach will be able to digest and process food properly; this will help you to get all the nutrients absorbed properly in blood and take all the benefits from it. Moreover, it will encourage you to avoid any kind of stomach problems, as your food is completely digested.

## Clean Blood Flow

During the fasting hours, as per schedule, you need to take liquids such as water or herbal teas that help you to clean up the blood. The more we drink water, the more we detox to finally get the blood purified. Moreover, it increases the blood flow to the whole body and in every organ as well. Better blood flow helps all the cells to receive the oxygenated blood and makes them healthy. Overall, you will get the best body health from the inside out. As a matter of fact, better blood flow helps the skin to breathe. It makes it tighten and bright as well; therefore, you will not only get a good body shape but radiant skin too.

Once you have better blood circulation to all the organs, providing them nutrients, proper rest, and exercise, it means that your overall health is getting better. It will make these organs function properly, and you will get the best lifestyle.

## Reduce Stress

Other than the body health benefits, this approach helps you to get rid of the psychological problems as well. An Intermittent Fasting eating pattern with balanced exercise can help you to deal with psychological stress problems. Good food and a healthy lifestyle make you relax and let out all the negativity that reduces stress and makes your life peaceful.

## Can Aid with Cancer

Several individuals have cancer cells yearly. The unchecked advancement of cells defines this horrible condition. Fasting has been disclosed to have some outstanding benefits when it pertains to your metabolic process, which may cause a lowered threat of cancer cells.

Some human research study studies disclose that cancer cells customers who fasted could lessen a few of the side results that include chemotherapy.

## Useful for the Mind

What is thought of fantastic for the body to benefit the mind likewise? Intermittent Fasting can help improve metabolic functions that are comprehended for aiding the mind to stay healthy. This could include assisting with insulin resistance, blood sugar level decrease, lowered inflammation, and oxidative tension. There have actually been some research study studies done on rats that demonstrate just how Intermittent Fasting can aid boost the development of brand-new afferent nerve cells, which improves the mind's function. Not eating can likewise assist in boosting the degrees of the brain-derived neurotrophic aspect. When the brain is lacking in this, it can activate depression together with a few other mental health issues.

## Autophagy

The cells in the body can start a waste removal when we go on a quick process that is recognized as autophagy, which involves the cells breaking down and metabolizing any kind of healthy proteins that cannot be made use of any longer. With an increased amount of autophagy, it might help protect the body from diseases such as Alzheimer's and also cancer cells.

## May Prevent Alzheimer

Alzheimer's is amongst the most common neurodegenerative illness. There is no cure for Alzheimer's, so the best step is to prevent it from happening as much as possible. One study that was carried out on rats showed that Intermittent Fasting could be able to delay the start of Alzheimer's disease or minimize its intensity. Some reports have really shown that a way of life modification that included some daily, or a minimum of regular, temporary fasts aided to improve the signs of Alzheimer's in 9 out of 10 clients. Pet research study studies additionally expose that this kind of fasting may aid in safeguarding against various other neurodegenerative diseases, such as Huntington's illness and Parkinson's.

Intermittent Fasting is a pattern, and research studies on ways it makes your body healthier are sensibly brand-new. It will take some time to examine all the advantages of recurring fasting.

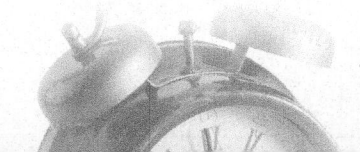

## CHAPTER 5

# Intermittent Fasting and the Fabulous 50s

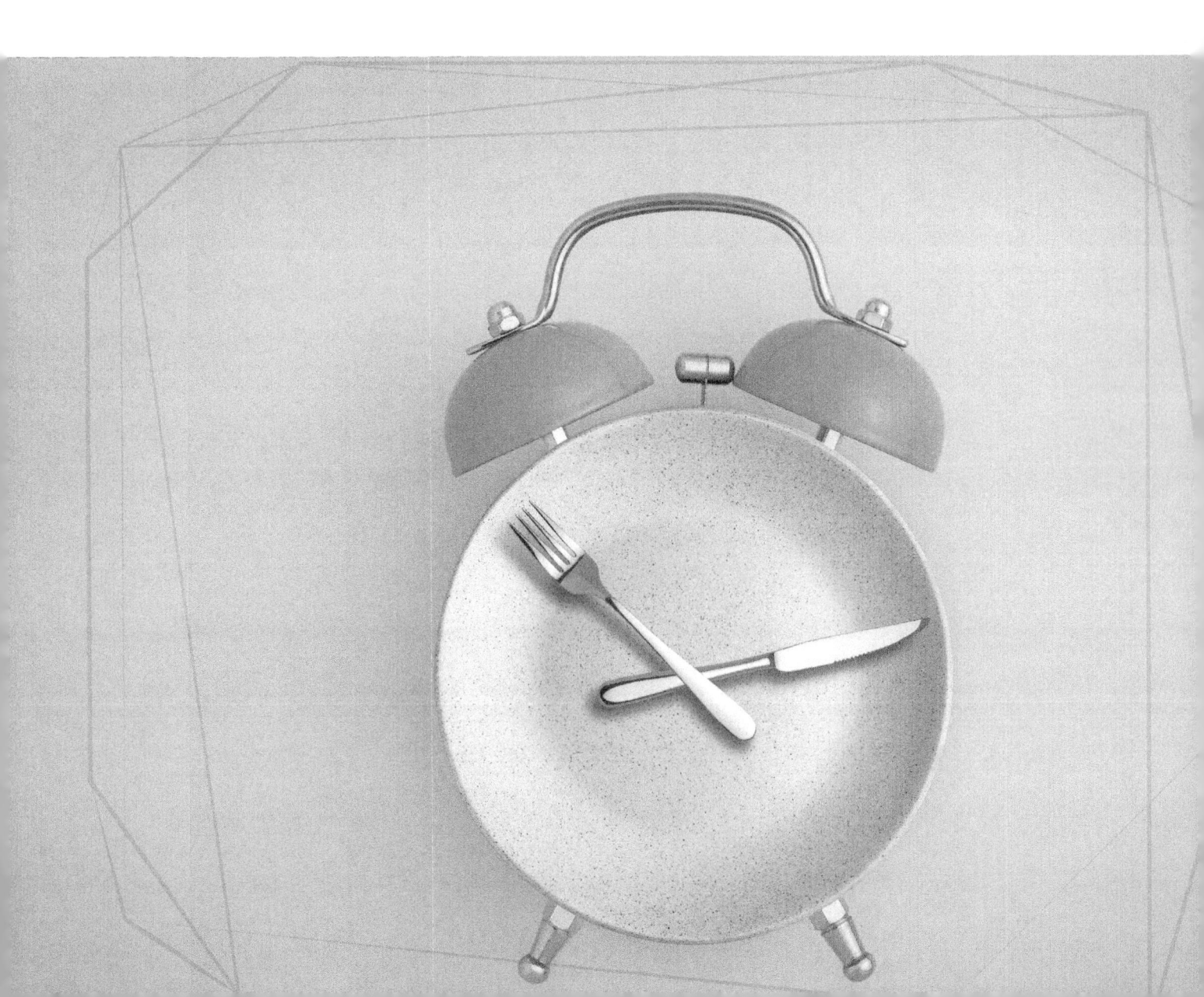

Intermittent Fasting is an effective way to naturally manage your menopausal symptoms and weight without the need for medication or crash dieting plans. There's no fad or crash dieting involved because you'll be eating certain foods in moderation and abstaining from food on a regular basis. Your body will be forced to use its stores of fat to burn for fuel, which promotes weight loss and prevents weight gain during menopause.

It also helps your body produce the right hormones for optimum health and wellness so you can enjoy the golden years of your life without all the symptoms associated with perimenopause and menopause.

## Mitigate the Effects Due To Body Changes After the 50s

After fifty, the internal systems of the body alter significantly, causing the body to burn calories less effectively than when you were younger. In addition, your body's nutritional requirements vary. Intermittent fasting helps us with the different issues related to these body changes. Said that let's go through at the main reasons why you should incorporate intermittent fasting after 50 into your life.

### You Start to Burn Fats and Calories More Efficiently

Instead of burning muscle and stored fat, the body burns calories via fat and stored food. When we are younger, our bodies use energy from protein stores first, then move on to burning also fat stores. Once fat stores are burned, the body starts burning muscle tissue as a means of survival. After 50, the body preferentially burns calories from fat stores and after age 60, protein is not burned as a primary source of energy.

### Hormone Levels Decrease After the Age of 50

The endocrine system, thyroid gland, and kidneys all produce hormones. The decrease in these hormones causes a decrease in hunger and a general lack of energy to do much of anything. In addition to these chemical changes in the body, changes also occur in the brain which controls appetite.

The brain begins to lower your need for food as it senses that food isn't necessary for survival so its signals aren't as pushy as before.

### Improved Metabolism Efficiency

Many people think their metabolisms have slowed down as they age, and they will never be able to lose weight or keep it off. However, research shows that a strict diet and exercise regime along with intermittent fasting can increase the metabolic rate by 5%, which can help you lose weight more easily than before.

### The Body Returns to its Normal Healing Status

Our bodies, in general, are always in the process of repairing themselves. As we start to age, our bodies must work harder to keep the body functioning at its peak performance level. Through fasting intermittently, the body's natural healing processes increase as less energy is spent on digesting food and more energy is available for repairing itself. Your immune system powers up to fight off infections as your body thinks it's starving.

### Brain Fog and Body Energy

Brain cells regenerate through intermittent fasting. This allows you to make better decisions and focus on the things that are important for you to do. You will find that your memory is sharper, and you are more apt to be able to think outside the box as your brain becomes more flexible with its ability to create new neural pathways. Your energy increases when you fast intermittently because your body has a chance to repair itself, restore energy, and build muscle mass which can lead to less fatigue over time.

### Storing Vitamins and Nutrients Will Be Easier for Your Body

Following sun exposure, the skin generates vitamin D, which is stored in the fatty layer under the skin. This vitamin is essential to building strong bones and muscles. The body holds on to calcium more tightly, making it less likely for you to lose bone and muscle mass.

### Increased Fitness Level

When you fast intermittently, you tend to find that with age, your stamina is higher, and your body gets stronger. You can do resistance training or any other type of physical activity as much as you want, and you won't feel tired or out of breath after the workout. Your muscles will repair themselves faster, so you aren't losing aerobics-based muscle mass as much as before.

### Feeling In a Good Shape and Mood

When you see results from fasting intermittently, you feel better about yourself on many levels.

## Intermittent Fasting and the Menopausal Effects

It must be said that a balanced diet has been carried out in life and there are no major weight fluctuations; this will no doubt be a factor that supports women who are going through menopause, but that it is not a sufficient condition to present with classic symptoms that are felt, which can be classified according to the period experienced. In fact, we can distinguish between the pre-menopausal phase, which lasts around 45 to 50 years, and is physiologically compatible with a drastic reduction in the production of the hormone estrogen (responsible for the menstrual cycle, which actually starts irregularly). This period is accompanied by a series of complex and highly subjective endocrine changes. Compare effectively: headache, depression, anxiety, and sleep disorders. When someone enters actual menopause, estrogen hormone production decreases even more dramatically, the range of the symptoms widens, leading to large amounts of the hormone, for example, to a certain class called catecholamine adrenaline.

The result of these changes is a dangerous heat wave, increased sweating, and the presence of tachycardia, which can be more or less severe. Although menopause causes major changes that greatly change a woman's body and soul, metabolism is one of the worst. In fact, during menopause, the absorption and accumulation of sugars and triglycerides changes, and it is easy to increase some clinical values such as cholesterol and triglycerides, which lead to high blood pressure or arteriosclerosis. In addition, many women often complain of disturbing circulatory disorders and local edema, especially in the stomach. It also makes weight gain easier, even though you haven't changed your eating habits.

### The Perfect Diet for Menopause

In cases where disorders related to the arrival of menopause become difficult to manage, drug or natural therapy under medical supervision may be necessary. The contribution given by a correct diet at this time can be considerable; in fact, given the profound variables that come into play, it is necessary to modify our food routine, both in order not to be surprised by all these changes and to adapt in the most natural way possible. In fact, they are also responsible for the classic hourglass shape of most women, which consists of depositing fat mainly on the hips, which begins to fail with menopause. As a result, we go from a gynoid condition to an android one, with an adipose increase localized on the belly. In addition, the metabolic rate of disposal is reduced; this means that even if you do not change your diet and eat the same quantities of food as you always have, you could experience weight gain, which will be more marked in the presence of bad habits or irregular diet. The digestion is also slower and intestinal function becomes more complicated. This further contributes to swelling as well as the occurrence of intolerance and digestive disorders which have never been disturbed before. Therefore, the beginning will be more problematic and difficult to manage during this period. The distribution of nutrients must be different: reducing the amount of low carbohydrate, which is always preferred not to be purified, helps avoid the peak of insulin and at the same time maintains stable blood sugar. These molecules are divided into three main groups, and the foods that contain them should never be missing on our tables: isoflavones, present mainly in legumes such as soy and red clover; lignans, of which flax seeds and oily seeds, in general, are particularly rich; coumestans, found in sunflower seeds, beans, and sprouts. A calcium supplementation will be necessary through cheeses such as parmesan, dairy products such as yogurt, egg yolk, some vegetables such as rocket, Brussels sprouts, broccoli, spinach, asparagus; legumes; dried fruit such as nuts, almonds, or dried grapes. Excellent additional habits that will help to regain well-being may be: limiting sweets to sporadic occasions, thus drastically reducing sugars (for example, by giving up sugar in coffee and getting used to drinking it bitterly); learn how to dose alcohol a lot (avoiding spirits, liqueurs, and aperitif drinks) and choose only one glass of good wine when you are in company, this because it tends to increase visceral fat which is precisely what is going to settle at the level abdominal. Clearly, even by eating lots of fruit, it is difficult to reach a high carbohydrate quota as in a traditional diet. However, a dietary plan to follow can be useful to have a more precise indication on how to distribute the foods. Obviously, one's diet must be structured in a personal way, based on specific metabolic needs and one's lifestyle.

## Does Intermittent Fasting Slow your Metabolism?

Many people think that skipping meals will make your body adapt to save energy by reducing its metabolic rate. It is well known that very long periods without food can cause a drop in metabolism. Moreover, studies have shown that fasting will improve the metabolism for short periods, not slow it down.

The definite answer is yes, but no more than other methods of weight loss. Nonetheless, if you can also maintain lean muscle, the effect on metabolism may be negligible. Nonetheless, relatively few studies focused specifically on intermittent fasting and metabolism and no long-term research. There is still a lot of that we don't know as such. But, even with the limitations of current research, it's clear that there's no need to avoid intermittent fasting due to potential metabolism impacts. Intermittent fasting indeed remains a powerful weight loss option, and many people find it effective. It is also worth noting that the weight-loss process itself can decrease metabolism. This pattern may be a significant reason why many people who have lost a great deal of weight end up. Your metabolic rate works like in a positive feedback loop—you eat more, you weigh more, you need more energy to keep that weight, your metabolic rate will be higher, and you need to eat more food to maintain the balance again. If you eat fewer calories than your TDEE due to fasting, dieting, or eating less, you will naturally lose some weight. If you repeat this pattern of putting less fuel into your body than its homeostatic set point, it will eventually down-regulate the requirements of the body for that energy that it does not get and become more preservative and more efficient with what it has. This will result in a slightly lower TDEE simply because your body needs less food. Image outcome for metabolism feedback loop Fasting down the metabolism is also mostly the result of actually eating less food or losing bodyweight, which will eventually decrease the body's caloric intake homeostasis as well. Funny enough, 48-hour fasting reportedly accelerates the metabolism by 3-14 percent. My theory is that the first days you're still running on your current TDEE when you start a fast, which causes a slight bump in energy expenditure, but after a while, you're going to lower it down as a natural defensive response. Fasting more than seven days will undoubtedly lower your demands on metabolism and protein. That is where your body goes into conservation mode and wants to keep as much energy as possible. Intermittent fasting can energize your metabolism to burn fat and help you lose weight, which gives your digestive system a rest. The trick is balancing fasting with a healthy diet and exercise and not taking it to extremes. If you have some health concerns, see your doctor before you try a fast one.

## How Does Intermittent Fasting Effect Metabolism?

This is a particular type of diet that, for some people at least, is effective for weight loss. An approach is essentially a form of dietary autophagy, and as a result, hunger is the focus. One of the most used types of intermittent fasting, for example, is the 16:8 diet, in which you only eat for 8 hours a day. While it may sound tough, many people find the food surprisingly easy. Yet, one of the questions most debated is: Does intermittent fasting slow metabolism? Short-Term Fasting and Metabolism The conventional idea is that you will slow down your metabolism by skipping food or fasting because your body has to make the things that it has to last longer. Cambridge Diet Feedback That is true in the long run. Further, if you dramatically reduce your calorie intake over an extended period or go a long time without food, this pattern makes sense for your metabolism. Metabolism is, after all, a reference to the speed with which the body burns fuel. If your reserves are low, it is not likely to be as fast. A short-term easy, though, is not the same thing. Indeed, some research has demonstrated that this practice can increase metabolism. One explanation for this may be that short-term fasting activates a norepinephrine hormone that can enhance fat burning. Also, many hormones have been related to short-term fasting. Insulin is one such example. Having too much insulin can make weight loss much more difficult because insulin tells the body to store fat effectively. Research shows that intermittent fasting can help lower levels of insulin. Another important hormone is the growth hormone of humans, which can aid fat loss. Research suggests that this hormone will increase dramatically during fasting and helps maintain muscle mass as well. Additionally, it is unlikely that the intermittent fasting approach will have the same impact as a very low-calorie diet. A 16:8 variation of the menu, for example, also means you're going a little longer without food than you would otherwise. Similarly, a variety of 5:2 only has two low-calorie days every week.

## Eliminates Wastes

"The Complete Idiot's Fasting Guide" states that one way to improve your metabolism by helping your body eliminate all the waste and toxins that accumulate from healthy eating and drinking is by fasting. Activates Human Growth Hormone, according to the Lean Look website, periodic 24-hour fasts are particularly beneficial since your body releases growth hormone after one has fasted for about 18 hours, which helps the body to burn fat and retain muscle.

## Regulates Digestion

This will affect your ability to metabolize your food and burn fat if your digestion is slow. "Fasting: The Ultimate Diet" states that intermittent fasts can control digestion and promote healthy bowel function, increasing metabolism.

## Improves Eating Habits

Daily fasts can change your attitude about food according to "Fasting: The Ultimate Diet." You will gain insight into your diet rather than being reliant on it and decide what your body requires for optimum work. Precise feeding energizes your metabolism. Slows Aging Fasting will delay the aging process by giving the body a break from regular digestion, according to "Fasting: The Ultimate Diet." This is important since one of the main effects of aging is a slower metabolism. The younger the body is, the quicker and more effective the fat-burning capacity of your metabolism.

## Each Body Is Different from the Others

Intermittent fasting is a weight-loss process. Further, as a result, it could potentially lead to both the loss of lean muscle and fat. This issue is popular across weight-loss approaches, particularly those that cut calories or protein intake drastically. For safety and metabolism, muscle mass is very significant. Specifically, having leaner muscle can play a key role in increasing metabolism and is also correlated with longevity. Yes, working to improve lean muscle is a critical piece of advice for improving metabolism. Doing so can involve getting more protein in your diet or working out (primarily through exercises for resistance). Multiple studies have now indicated that intermittent fasting impacts lean body mass similarly to calorie restriction. Furthermore, this means that intermittent fasting can have a negative effect on your body composition but nothing more than a simple limit on calories. Through that process, intermittent fasting may potentially reduce metabolism.

# CHAPTER 6

# Intermittent Fasting Possible Side Effects

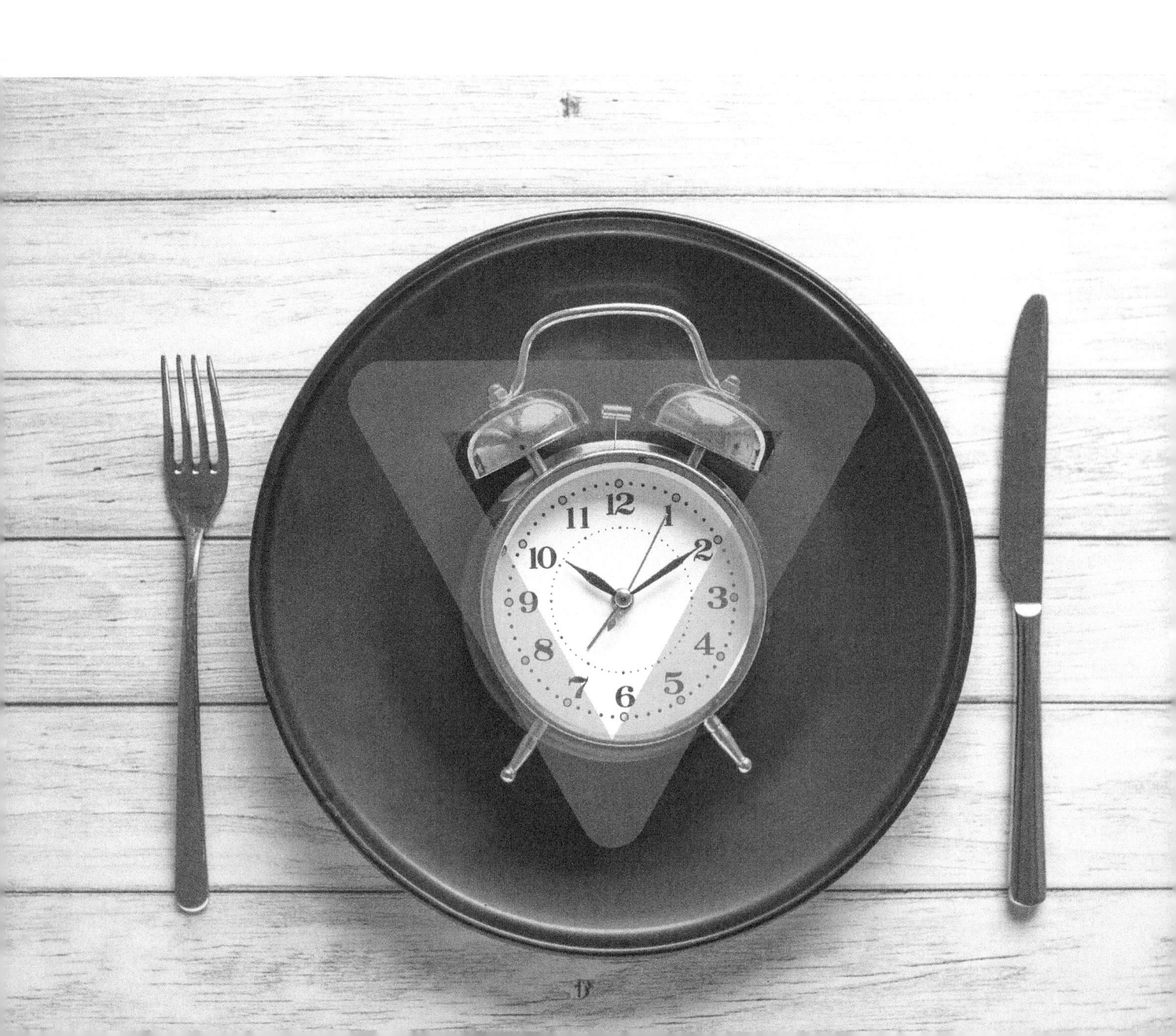

Although intermittent fasting has many advantages and benefits, there are likewise some possible negative effects to be considered.

Any individual who is going to begin a regular fasting eating pattern at any point shortly has to know both the positive and negative effects of fasting and afterward choose either it's advantageous for your body or not.

## Anxiety Attacks

A potential side effect of detoxing through Intermittent Fasting is the potential for an anxiety attack. This can happen when you are withholding food for an extended period of time, especially if you are new to Intermittent Fasting.

An anxiety attack may come upon you because you feel that you are not getting enough nutrition or missing your usual feeding times.

## Digestive Distress

Since Intermittent Fasting has a detoxing component to it, you may experience digestive distress during your first few experiences. This is due to your body flushing out much of the residual matter in your body in addition to simply excreting whatever is still leftover in the digestive tract.

While this is normal to a certain extent, care should be taken if you happen to experience severe diarrhea. This may be especially true if you jump into a fasting period after overeating the preceding day. As long as it isn't anything that you feel abnormal, you can attribute it to the detoxing process. However, if symptoms do not subside, then you may need to seek medical attention at once.

## You Might Struggle to Maintain Blood Sugar Levels

Although the Intermittent Fasting diet tends to improve blood sugar levels in most people, this is not always true for everyone. Some people who are adopting the Intermittent Fasting eating pattern may find that their ability to maintain a healthy blood sugar level is compromised.

The reason why this happens varies. For some people, not eating frequently enough may encourage this to happen. For others, transitioning too quickly or taking on too intense of a fasting cycle too soon can result in a shock to the body that causes a strange fluctuation in blood sugar levels.

## You Might Experience Hormonal Imbalances

A certain degree of fasting, especially when you build up to it, can support you in having healthier hormone levels. However, for some people, Intermittent Fasting may lead to an unhealthy imbalance of hormones. This can result in a whole slew of different hormone-based symptoms, such as headaches, fatigue, and even menstrual problems in women.

Again, the reason for the hormonal imbalance varies. For some people, particularly those who are already at risk of experiencing hormonal imbalances, Intermittent Fasting can trigger these imbalances to take place. For others, it could go back to what they are consuming during the eating windows. Eating meals that are not rich in nutrients and vitamins can result in you not having enough nutrition to support your hormonal levels.

If you begin experiencing hormonal imbalances when you eat the Intermittent Fasting Diet, it is essential that you stop and consult your doctor right away. Discovering where the shortcomings are and how you can correct them is vital. Having imbalanced hormones for too long can lead to diseases and illnesses that require constant life-long attention.

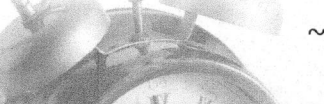

## Headaches

A decrease in your blood sugar level and the release of stress hormones by your brain as a result of going without food are possible causes of headaches during the fasting window. Problems may also be a clear message from your body telling you that you are very low on water and getting dehydrated. This may happen if you are completely engrossed in your daily activities and you forget to drink the required amount of water your body needs during fasting.

To handle headaches, ensure you stay well hydrated throughout your fasting window. Keep in mind that exceeding the required amount of water per day may also result in adverse effects. Reducing your stress level can also keep headaches away.

## Cravings

During your fasting periods, you might find that you have higher levels of desire than usual. This often happens because you are telling yourself that you cannot have any food, so suddenly, you start craving many different foods. This is because all you are thinking about is food. As you think about food, you will begin to think about the different types of food you like and want. Then, the cravings start.

Early on, you may also find yourself craving more sweets or carbs because your body is searching for an energy hit through glucose. While you do not want to have excessive levels of sugar during your eating window, as this is bad for blood sugar, you can always have some. The ability to satisfy your cravings is one of the benefits of eating a diet that is not as restrictive as some other foods are.

## Low Energy

A feeling of lethargy is not uncommon during fasting, especially at the start. This is your body's natural reaction to switching its source of energy from glucose in your meals to fat stored in your body. So, expect to feel a little less energized in your first few weeks of starting with Intermittent Fasting. To troubleshoot the feeling of lethargy, try as much as possible to stay away from overly strenuous activities. Keep things low-key. Spending more time sleeping or just relaxing is another proper way to ensure that your energy reserves are not depleted too quickly. The first few weeks are not the time to test your limits or push yourself.

## Foul Mood

You may find yourself being on edge during fasting, even if you are someone who is naturally predisposed to being good-natured. The reason for the feeling of edginess is straightforward. You are hungry, yet you won't eat, and you are struggling to keep your cravings in check; plus, you may already be feeling tired and sluggish. Add all of these to the internal hormone changes due to the sharp decline in your blood sugar levels, and it's no wonder why you may be in such a foul mood. Tempers can easily flare up, and you may be quick to become irritated. This is normal when beginning a fasting lifestyle.

## Excess Urination

Fasting tends to make you visit the bathroom more frequently than usual. This is an expected side effect since you are drinking more water and other liquids than before. Avoiding water to reduce the number of times you use the bathroom is not a good idea at all, no matter how you look at it. Cutting down water intake while you are fasting will make your body become dehydrated very quickly. If that happens, losing weight will be the least of your problems. Whatever you do, do not avoid drinking water when you are fasting. Doing that is paving the way for a humongous health disaster waiting to happen. You don't want to do that.

## Heartburn, Bloating, and Constipation

Your stomach is responsible for producing stomach acid, which is used to break down food and trigger the digestion process. When you eat frequent meals, huge meals, regularly, your body is used to producing high amounts of stomach acid to break down your food. As you transition to a fasting diet, your stomach has to get used to not producing as much stomach acid.

You might also notice an increase in constipation and bloating. People who eat regularly consume high amounts of fiber and proteins that support a healthy digestion process. When you switch to the Intermittent Fasting cycle, you can still eat a high volume of fiber and protein.

However, early on, you might find that you forget to. As you discover the proper eating habits that work for you, it may take some time for you to get used to finding ways to work in enough fiber and protein to keep your digestion flowing.

Heartburn may not be a widespread adverse effect, but it does sometimes occur in some individuals. Your stomach produces highly concentrated acids to help break down the foods you consume. But when you are fasting, there is no food in your stomach to be broken down, even though acids have already been produced for that purpose. This may lead to heartburn.

Bloating and constipation usually go hand in hand and can be very discomforting to individuals who suffer from it due to fasting.

Heeding the advice to drink adequate amounts of water usually keeps bloating and constipation in check. Heartburn typically resolves itself quickly, but you can take an antacid tablet or 2 if it persists. You may also consider eating fewer spicy foods when you break your fast.

## You Might Start Feeling Cold

As you begin to adjust to your Intermittent Fasting Diet, you might find that your fingers and toes get quite cold. This happens because blood flow towards your fat stores is increasing, so blood flow to your extremities reduces slightly. This supports your body in moving fat to your muscles so that it can be burned as fuel to keep your energy levels up.

## You Might Find Yourself Overeating

The chances for overeating during the break of the fast are high, especially for beginners. Understandably, you will feel starving after going without food for longer than you are used to. This hunger causes some people to eat hurriedly and surpass their standard meal size and average caloric intake. For others, overeating may be a result of an uncontrollable appetite. Hunger may push some people to prepare too much food for breaking their fast, and if they don't have a grip on their desire, they will continue to eat even when they are satiated. Overeating or binging when you break your fast will make it difficult to reach your optimal health and fitness goal.

## Hunger

People who start Intermittent Fasting may initially feel quite hungry. This is especially common if you are the type of person who tends to eat regular meals daily.

If you start feeling hungry, you can choose to wait it out if you have an eating window right around the corner. However, if there is a more extended waiting period or you are feeling starving, you should eat. Feeling hungry to the point that it becomes uncomfortable or distracting is not helpful and will not support you in successfully taking on the Intermittent Fasting Diet. This is a pronounced side effect of going without food for longer than you are accustomed to.

## CHAPTER 7

# How to Stick Into Intermittent Fasting

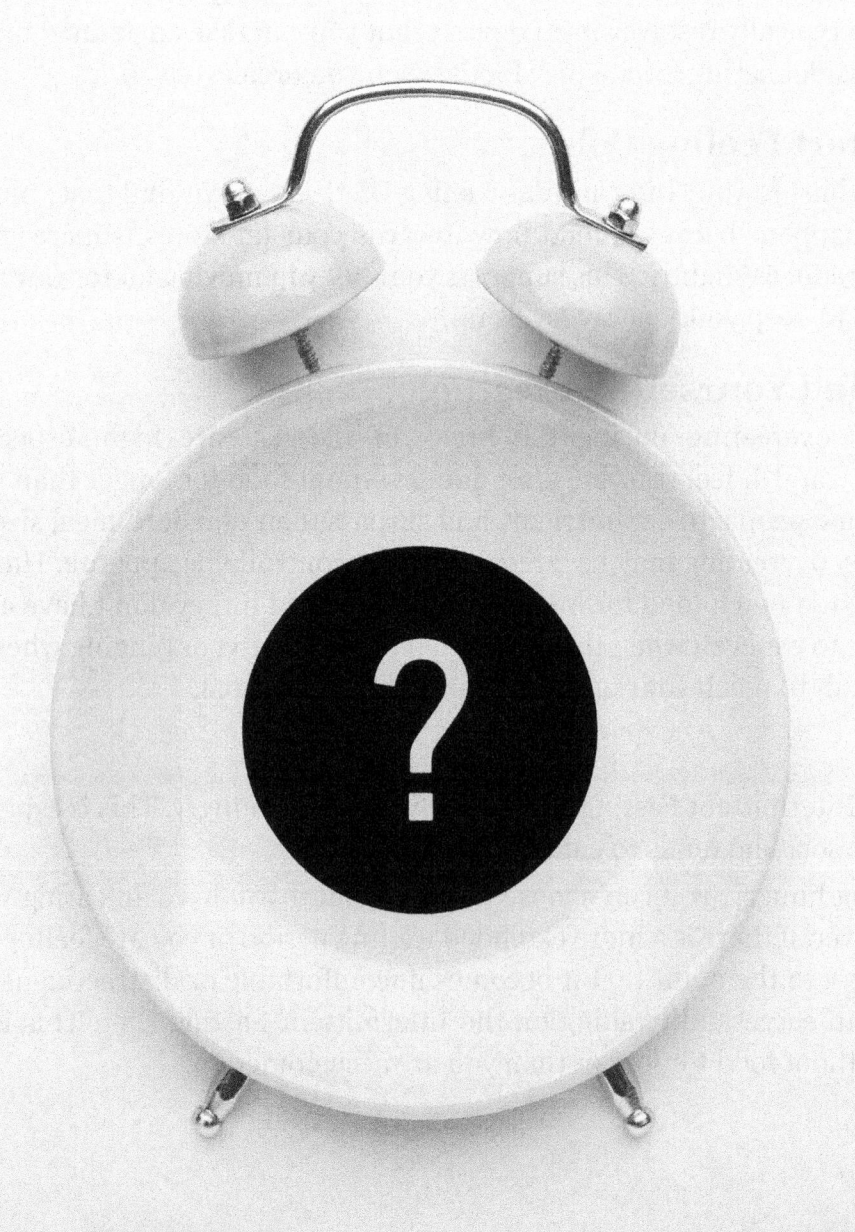

Sticking to a fasting routine can be tricky for anyone. This is why tips are helpful. They can help you stay on track when your motivation ebbs and the weight loss plateau begins. Here are some of the most important tips to keep in mind while fasting:

## Plan Healthy

Make sure to plan ahead. You must have healthy food available when hunger pangs hit. You should try to avoid hunger by keeping a supply of healthy snacks in the house. This will help you avoid unnecessary snacking on unhealthy foods during your fast.

If you are not used to fasting, it is better to start with short fasting periods before extending them to longer ones. When starting, try skipping breakfast for a few days in a row. Drink lots of water and avoid coffee and other caffeinated beverages during this time period as they can increase your appetite.

## Rise Early

Fasting can be more natural when done when the day is young because energy levels are at their peak, and the chances of feeling hungry are lower. If you skip breakfast, you can stop eating until lunchtime.

Fasting becomes a lot easier if you are busy with work or other activities. When fasting is done while doing something else, the hunger pangs would be less intense.

A good strategy for fasting is to exercise first thing in the morning before having breakfast. This will start your day with energy and make it easier to deal with hunger pangs. You should avoid doing vigorous activities after exercise, however, as they can increase your appetite and make it harder to stick to fasting. Exercise also makes you hungry after it's over, so be prepared for that. On days when you cannot exercise, try walking or performing light exercises instead, which would still help reduce hunger pangs.

## Exercise

Exercising would help keep hunger pangs at bay during fasting. You might also feel more energetic when you exercise, which can make you feel better and overall more motivated to stick to your fasting routine.

## Keep The Focus on Health Benefits

One of the reasons that people fail to stick with fasting is because they get easily lured by the taste of forbidden foods. With this in mind, it is important to remind yourself of your long-term goals whenever you get tempted to have a snack. Remind yourself why you went on a fast in the first place and how improved health will benefit your life in the long run.

## Nutritious Meals Ahead of Time

Before starting your fast, have a meal made of foods that are rich in protein but low in calories. Also, ensure that you include plenty of vegetables in your meal.

## Don't Skip Meals

Fasting is not something you do forever. Like any other diet, it takes time, and the number of days to stay on it should be counted from the day you started. It is advisable not to skip meals: if you do so, your body will start craving food in order to take care of its needs, and this might add extra pressure on your willpower which can possibly lead you to quit fasting altogether.

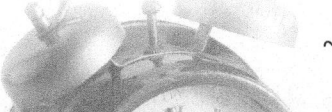

## Prep Your Meals in Advance

You should prepare your meals in advance. If you are planning to fast for a longer period, try to have enough food at home for one week. This will help you avoid unhealthy snacking, which would otherwise lead you to overeat later and undo the effects of your fasting.

## Maintain Healthy Records

It is important that you keep a record of your weight and measurements of your body so that you can see improvement every time you go on a fast. You should also be able to see the health benefits from the weight loss by noting down the number on the scale every day or at least know how much healthier your body is becoming by looking at the photos of yourself before and after the fast.

## Give Yourself Time to Adjust Them

It is important to give yourself time to adjust after you have started fasting. During the first week or 2, the hunger pangs and cravings can be intense. You should keep on with your fast even though you have a hard time because it will help you adjust when the hunger pangs and cravings have subsided.

## Stick a Routine

There are many different kinds of fasting routines. Which one you choose is up to you but it is important that you stick to it. This will help your body get used to the fasting routine and also help your mind accept and understand the importance of fasting.

## Stay Positive

It is crucial that you do not make fasting a negative experience because this might lead you to give up before achieving your goals. Instead, think of it as a positive thing for you and keep telling yourself how beneficial fasts can be for your health and well-being.

## Drink Lots of Water

This might seem a little strange, but drinking water even if you don't feel thirsty can help to keep hunger pangs at bay. You can also use the time to drink more water since this is also part of a fasting routine.

Moreover, drinking lots of water can help you feel full even if you are not eating so much food. It can also help flush out toxins from your body and keep your digestive system as healthy as possible.

## Discipline Yourself

Reaching goals requires discipline and self-control. Fasting will test those 2 things in you, but it is important that you do not give up no matter what kind of challenge it becomes. This may be difficult, but it will pay off in the long run when you achieve your goals in a shorter period of time with less effort and greater success.

# CHAPTER 8

# Mistakes to Avoid

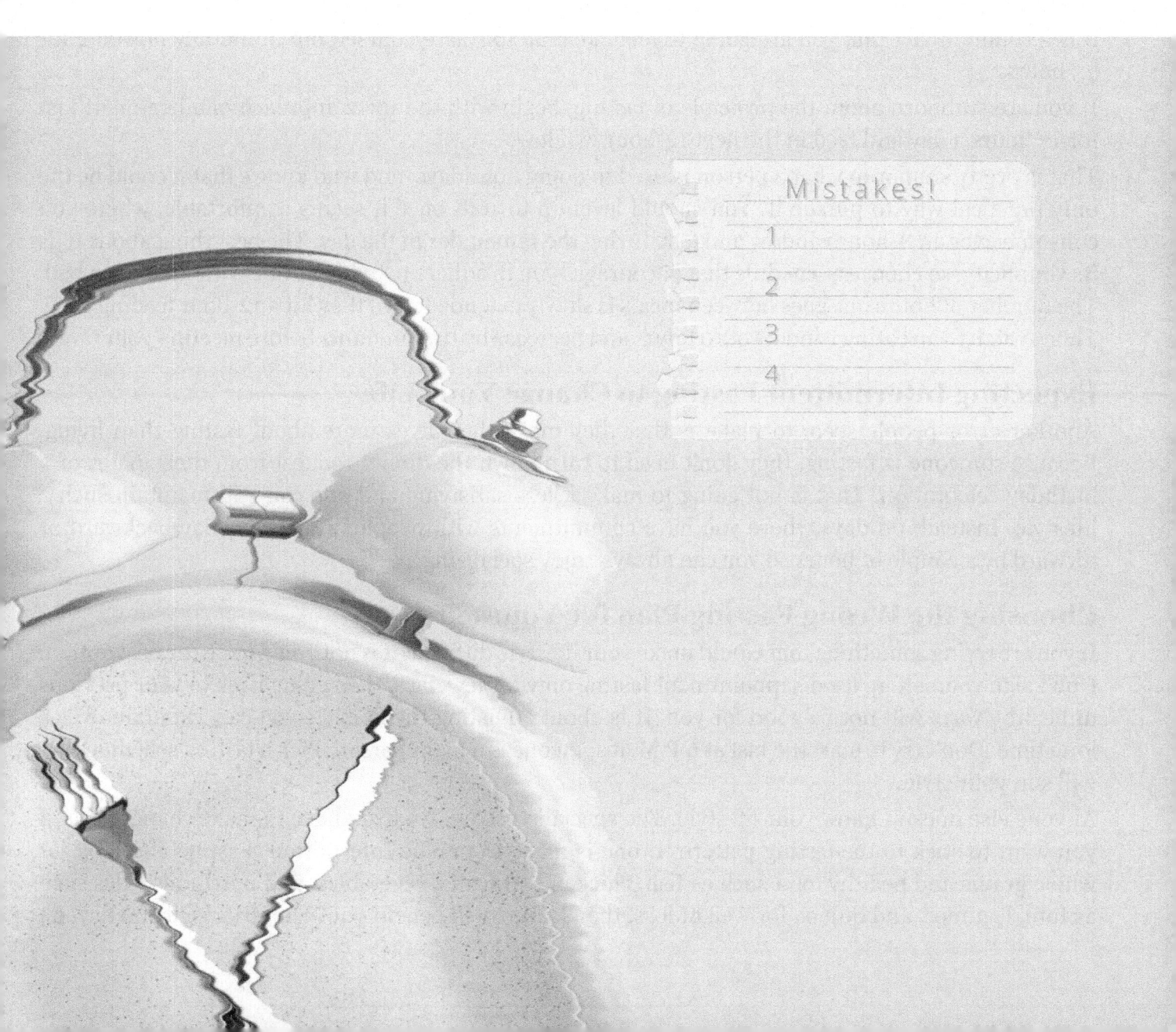

When it comes to Intermittent Fasting for beginners, it is necessary to avoid these misconceptions and mistakes no matter your age.

### Rushing into Intermittent Fasting

You are more likely to get hungry all the time and discouraged if you are regularly eating every 3–4 hours and then unexpectedly shrink your mealtime to only 8 hours. According to some experts, any individuals will stop Intermittent Fasting if they start fasting for many hours without a transition time from a prior eating style.

Instead, ease slowly into fasting. If you are going for the 16:8 technique, progressively increase the period between meals so you can operate within 12 hours comfortably. Then, add multiple hours a day before you get to the 8-hour window.

There are levels of Intermittent Fasting. The primary factor most diets don't harvest benefits is their drastic deviation from our normal, usual eating habits. Sometimes, it can seem not easy to sustain. You think about it if someone is new to IF, then they are used to eating every 2 hours, you are going to feel very uncomfortable during the long hours of fasting. It is normal to have a transition time, but it should feel better.

A remarkably strong communicator is the body itself. If it feels like trouble, it will let you know. And it is a common fact that you are going to feel like crap to starve yourself out of literally nowhere for 23 hours.

If you are stubborn about the principle of fasting, begin with the 12:12 approach of a beginner: fast for 12 hours a day and feed in the next 12-hour window.

That is pretty similar to what a person is used to doing nowadays, and who knows that it could be the only practical way to pursue it. You should level up to 16:8 once it seems comfortable, where you consume over an 8-hour window and fast during the remainder of the day. The best thing about IF is its simplicity, so choose a schedule that encourages you to adhere to a time frame without feeling bad. The number of hours one goes between meals is slowly extended until they hit a 12-hour feeding time. Then switch to an eating window of 10 hours and decrease by tiny amounts before meeting your target.

## Expecting Intermittent Fasting to Change Your Life

Another error people seem to make is that they make their lives more about fasting than living. Because someone is fasting, they don't need to turn down the dinner request from their mates or a birthday celebration. That is not going to make it less satisfying and one can still maintain such a lifestyle. Instead, on days where you have commitments with people, move your day backward or forward by a couple of hours so you can always enjoy socializing.

## Choosing the Wrong Fasting Plan for Yourself

If you are trying something that would make your lifestyle difficult, it is not going to be the best option. Don't sign yourself up for disappointment fasting only for few days, then going back to your previous unhealthy ways will not be good for you. It is about adjusting the lifestyle you can maintain over a long time. Don't try to start the fast at 6 P.M. if someone is a night person. Pick a fasting schedule that will suit your style.

Anyone else doesn't know your lifestyle. The specialist is you. And you have to make changes that if you want to stick to the fasting pattern. If one is ready to pursue Intermittent Fasting and look for whole grains and healthy food such as fish, chicken and fruits, vegetables, and nutritious sides such as tofu, legumes, and quinoa for weight loss, then fasting will benefit you. The issue is, if you haven't picked the right IF strategy, it will not give you success. Like if you are a committed gym-goer 6 days each week, the perfect schedule might not be too fast entirely on 2 of those days.

## Not Drinking Enough and Drinking the Wrong Stuff

An Intermittent Fasting error to avoid is consuming the wrong drinks and not drinking sufficiently while fasting. Even if it is calorie-free, you don't want to consume something that is overly sweetened. Since it also has a detrimental impact on insulin levels and will stimulate your appetite and make you want to snack.

When fasting, aim to stick to water, pure tea, or black coffee. If one doesn't drink sufficiently, it may also cause dehydration, contributing to headaches, muscle cramps, and exacerbating hunger pangs.

## Overeating when Fasting Ends

Overeating after completing the fast is another famous error. When a fast ends, it may be simple to overeat just because one may feel ravenous, or people justify themselves because they made up for missed calories, which is why they overeat.

But if you are fasting for weight reduction especially, this may turn out badly and even trigger some issues, including stomach aches. Prepare your meals beforehand; when your fast finishes, cook a nutritious recipe that is available for you and ensure that you consume whole foods wherever possible, including healthy carbohydrates such as seafood, vegetables, lean protein, and whole grains.

## Eating Too Much in the Fasting Window

Most of the time, people want to pursue Intermittent Fasting is because it involves eating fewer calories; it means they also will have less time to eat. In the duration of the fasting window, though, certain individuals will consume their normal amount of calories. This will imply you are not going to lose weight. Don't consume the normal intake of calories in the window. Rather, when one breaks the fast, expect to consume about 1,200–1,500 calories. If it is 4, 6, 8 hours, how many meals one can consume would depend on the duration of the fasting window.

If you need to overeat and are in a condition of starvation, reconsider the strategy you want to adopt or relax off the IF for a day to regroup and then get back on board.

## Forcing it on yourself

Forcing the body to fast is yet another error. It is necessary to note that it is not for everybody to start Intermittent Fasting. It is all right to re-assess if this is the best strategy for you. Yes, some say that our bodies will cope quite frequently with hunger, but that doesn't imply that it is the best thing for everyone to do right now.

Not all bodies are developed for intermittent fasting. Ask yourself this easy question if intermittent fasting seems like a relentless challenge and emotional drain: Is the compromised standard of life worth it?

## Not Paying Attention to the Nutrient Quality of the Foods

When following Intermittent Fasting, people often rely on fast foods when they simply concentrate on what to eat more than what they should consume. Instead of keeping a well-balanced diet, if you continue with refined foods, you should not anticipate Intermittent Fasting to achieve your fitness goals. By adopting nutritious foods steadily, aim to adjust your lifestyle along with your meal routine progressively.

## Restricting the Food Intake too much

You have got to note that fasting is not for starving. Our bodies need fuel to move around, work properly, think straight, and converse naturally, and that fuel comes from food. It takes a toll on daily life to limit your food consumption so much, and that is not the main concern of what fasting is all about.

The "what" is overlooked in favor of the "when." IF is a time-centered eating pattern, and most schedules don't include any clear guidelines during the feeding window for the kinds of food to consume. Although this is not an accessible invitation for French fries, beer, and milkshakes, to thrive. Fasting is not magic. In addition to certain minor physiological effects, the main influence on weight reduction is that you minimize the hours of feeding and the number of calories you eat.

Sadly, by selecting the wrong types of foods, you cannot easily reverse the influence. During the feeding hours, change your mindset from a "treating yourself" attitude to one that centers around consuming the most nutrient-packed, nourishing meals you can find. To better fill yourself up and carry you during the fasting process, we suggest the following:

- Make sure any meal or snack contains a mix of fiber, protein, and good fats.
- Cook all the meals at home and try not to eat takeout's or in restaurants.
- Pay attention to nutrition labels and make sure to not consume forbidden ingredients like modified palm oil, corn syrup, high fructose.
- Try to consume low sodium and beware of added sugar.
- Do not eat processed foods and home cook whole foods.
- Add fiber, good fats, and lean proteins to your plate.

# CHAPTER 9

# Exercise and Intermittent Fasting

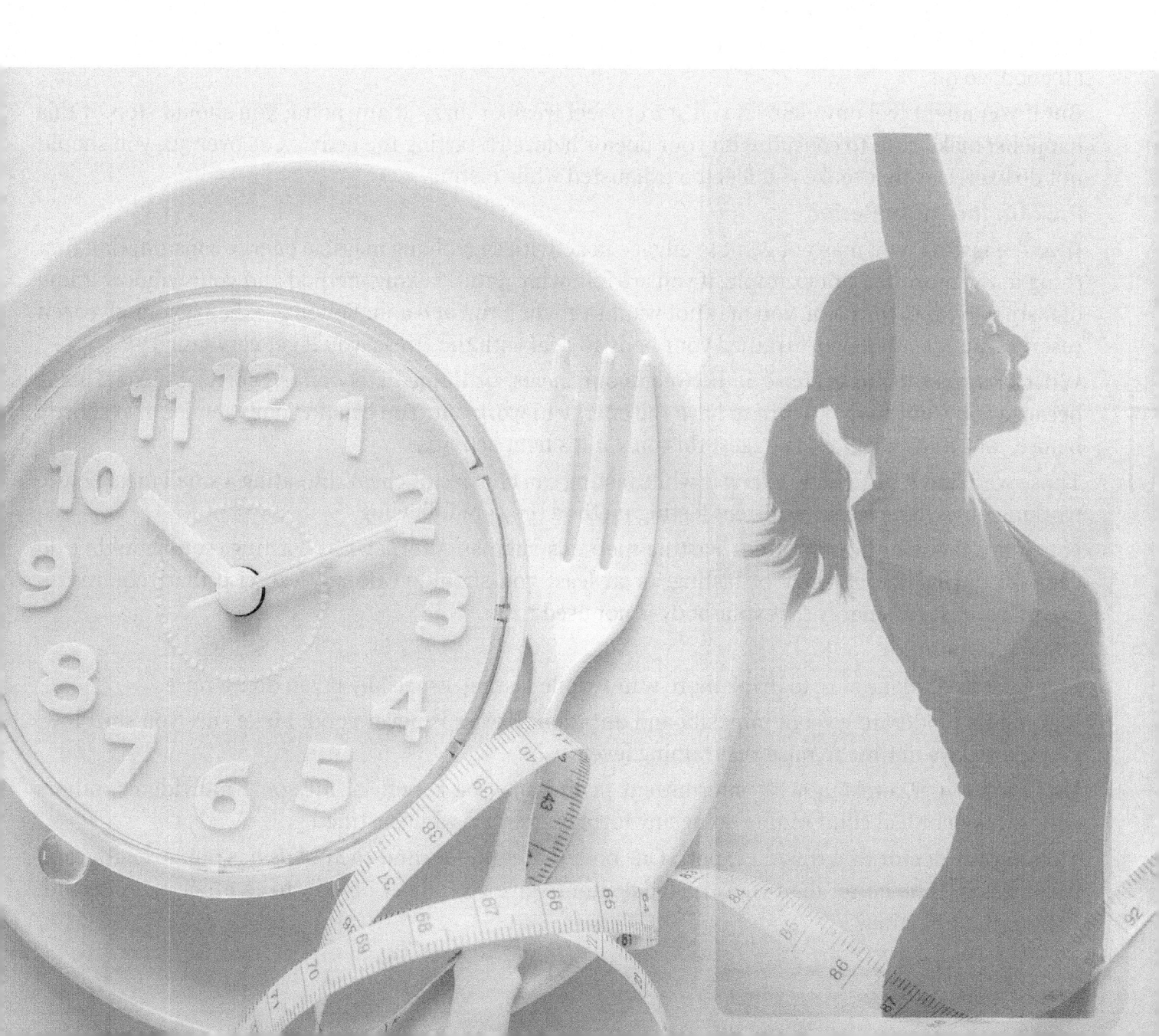

# How to Exercise Safely During Intermittent Fasting

Physical activity is the third and final component of the weight-loss triad, but it is no less important. Exercising increases blood flow, activates endorphins after and during workouts, and can aid in calorie burn. The amount of calories you burn is determined by the form, length, and strength of the exercise. However, this is usually a small amount compared to the number of calories burned by your basal metabolic rate.

Intermittent fasting will help control your energy levels by depleting available glycogen reserves, causing your body to burn fat if it isn't already doing so. Do you recall those old-school fitness videos where everybody was all about "feeling the burn"? Exercising only burns fat in a very small percentage of cases. In reality, fat is only burned after glycogen stores have been depleted (which takes a while).

Said that, If you are doing Intermittent Fasting and you are over 50, it's completely fine doing exercise. I suggest only paying a little more attention to a few simple aspects when doing exercise during fasting.

### Always Listen to Your Body

Your body is the best indicator to understand if you are doing well. How you feel when you begin to exercise is an excellent indication of whether you're ready for it. Do you feel exhausted and unable to continue, or do you feel you can go on?

If you feel that your body is reacting well without excessive fatigue and you are enjoying the activity, all good, go on.

But if you might feel unwell, or if you start to feel weak or dizzy at any point, you should stop. If this happens, make sure to consult with your doctor before restarting the activity, as over 50, you should not do exercises that make you feel too exhausted while fasting.

### Pick Up the Right Period

If you're fasting, you may not want to engage in activities involving massive energy consumption first thing in the morning. For example, if you are following a 16:8 fasting method and your window frame of fasting is 7 p.m to 11 a.m, you may not want to go for a run at 8 a.m. You may exhaust your glycogen reserves, and if you haven't trained your body to deal with the stress, you'll get very hungry.

What I suggest it's to exercise in between your meals, or immediately after your last meal. This is because you want to make sure to have the energy to work out. You can do your exercise also shortly before your first meal, but I suggest this only if it's light activity.

Those who find it difficult to exercise while fasting can choose to "cheat" by eating a small meal before working out, whatever intermittent fasting method they are following.

If you are following Intermittent Fasting methods such as Alternat-Day Fasting, you shouldn't do exercise during the 24-hour of fasting, or at least you shouldn't do any exercise that requires an excessive waste of energy that your body is not used to.

### Other Suggestion

Stay hydrated. Make sure to drink more water while fasting, especially if you do exercise.

Maintain a moderate level of intensity and duration. Excess is never good. Make sure you start low; you are always in time to raise the training level.

Don't force it. Exercising with intermittent fasting may be beneficial for some individuals; others simply may not feel comfortable doing any form of exercise while fasting.

Talk to your doctor or a trusted expert. Our bodies are unique, and each of us has our strengths and weaknesses. Who better than your trusted doctor to give you advice on how to combine exercise with Intermittent Fasting?

To conclude I would like to clarify that these indications are clearly addressed to beginners. Those women who are not used to doing physical exercise but would like to start doing it, or they are doing it lightly, in this particular moment of their life.

If you're an experienced athlete or are used to an advanced level of exercise, you've probably already talked to a specialist about combining your physical activity with the Intermittent Fasting eating pattern. If you haven't already done so, I suggest you do it.

## Light Activities

### Walking

This is a very easy form of exercise and can be done by anyone. It can also be done anywhere, including at your home.

### Yoga

Yoga is a great way to relax and get in some exercise at the same time. You are in control of how intense this form of exercise can be and with over 300 different types it allows everyone to find their perfect fit. It has been known to reduce symptoms such as anxiety, depression, stress levels, fatigue, and insomnia when practiced regularly.

### Tai Chi

Tai Chi is a form of moving meditation; it uses slow and gentle movements to relax and calm your mind. It can also ease symptoms such as depression, anxiety, and stress. The movements are very gentle, so even people with limited mobility can take part in this practice.

### Dancing

Yes, you read that right; dancing is a great form of exercise that has many benefits, such as improved brain function, coordination, muscle tone, and positive moods. Just make sure you choose a form of dance that you enjoy, as this will motivate you to keep going back for more!

### Aerobics

This involves rhythmic movements combined with deep breathing that improves strength, endurance, and cardiovascular fitness. There are many different types of aerobics, some of which are cardio dance, basic step aerobics, kickboxing, and Zumba.

### Circuit Training

This type of exercise involves a series of exercises that work for different muscle groups at the same time. It is a great way to burn fat and tone muscles together; it is also great for the fitness conscience as it takes the hard work out of getting in shape! It can be done anywhere from a park bench to your own home.

## Moderate Activities

### Pilates

Pilates is a great form of exercise that has many benefits, such as increased flexibility, strength, and endurance. It involves a series of mat exercises combined with stretching that makes the whole process easier for both you and your muscles. Pilates is a great form of exercise for the elderly as it can help prevent loss of muscle tone.

### Swimming

Swimming is a great way to keep yourself fit, and improves flexibility, strength, and endurance while helping to burn calories in the process.

It does not involve any impact, so it is great for people with joint problems. It also helps improve your cardiovascular fitness and helps tone your muscles.

**Running**

Running is a very popular form of exercise that is enjoyed by many. It offers many physical benefits, such as improved lung capacity, heart health, and weight loss. It can also have mental benefits, such as stress levels being reduced when you exercise regularly.

**Rowing**

This form of exercise is very popular among the elderly as it is low-impact and can help to prevent further loss of muscle tone. It also helps improve your cardiovascular health and can reduce stress levels.

**Bicycling**

Bicycling has many benefits, such as improving mental health and reducing stress levels. It also improves your balance and decreases the risk of falling. This form of exercise can be done anywhere you like, from your home to the beach or park!

*30-Day Meal Plan*

# CHAPTER 10

# FAQ & Myth to Dissolve

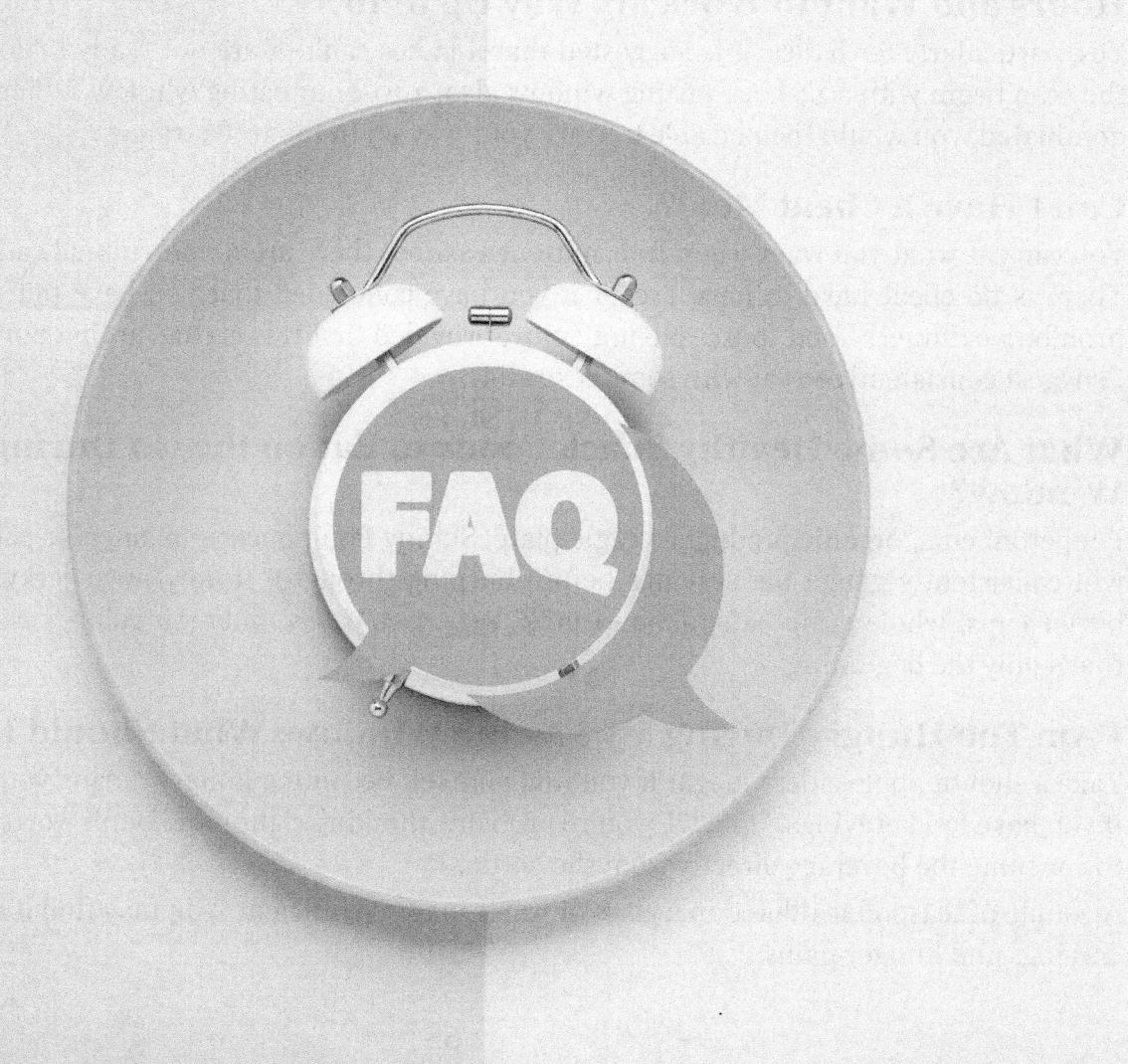

## Can I Drink Coffee or Tea When I'm fasting?
Truly, you can have black coffee, water, and plain tea during your fasting window

## Can I Add Cream/Sugar/Milk to My Coffee?
The objective of fasting isn't to add Calories, so the appropriate response is no; you ought not to add anything to your espresso. Nonetheless, I have known about cases in which intermittent fasters add under 50 Calories to their coffee. T

hey have professed to be effective with IF; I have heard that it doesn't influence their abstained state; however, remember all people are most certainly not the same. I would not prescribe adding anything to your coffee, yet if adding something to your espresso makes this a good chance for the objective you have for yourself, at that point, check it out.

## Does Intermittent Fasting Work Well with Veganism, Paleo, Keto, Vegetarianism, or Any Other Styles of Eating?
Indeed, the magnificence of Intermittent Fasting is that it tends to be joined with any way of eating except if coordinated by a clinical expert.

You can transform your way of eating into the any Intermittent Fasting technique effortlessly, as this change does not limit or express the style/sorts of food you eat; it is explicitly founded on the condition of your eating.

## Is There an Alternative to the 16:8 Method If I Cannot Initially Fast 16 Hours and Want to Work My Way Up to 16?
Yes, particularly for ladies, it is suggested that if ladies can't or are not ready to do a 16-hour quick, they can begin with a 14-hour fasting window also, a 10-hour eating window. When the 14 hours are dominated, you would then be able to work your way up to the 16:8 strategy.

## Can I Have a Cheat Meal?
You can eat what you want when Intermittent Fasting; there are no nutritional category limitations. There is no cheat meal to have except if you have concluded that you have put yourself on some prohibitive dinners/food sources to not enjoy; provided that this is true, at that point truly, however, I suggest consistently to eat with some restraint.

## What Are Some Healthy Snack Foods to Eat on the Go During My Feeding Window?
Pepperoni cuts, organic products, veggie plate, Skinny Pop popcorn in singular packs (except if you will consistently gauge the servings before burning-through), turkey/meat jerky, singular peanut butter cups, whole grain oats, almond milk, eggs, rice cakes, nuts (singular packs), hummus, and that's only the beginning.

## I Am Too Hungry During My Fasting Window; What Should I Do?
Take a shot of apple cider vinegar if you find yourself becoming hungry during your fasting hours or if you have food cravings. "Eew!?!" you're probably thinking right now. Don't worry; you do not need to consume the beverage directly from the bottle.

A couple of teaspoons diluted in a glass of water may be sufficient. You may find it reduces your food cravings and hunger pains.

If you really can't with apple cider vinegar, especially at the beginning, I suggest eating some walnuts, just to get used to it, though!

## Why Am I Not Losing Fat Faster, Like Other People Are?

It is without a doubt a mix of not eating the appropriate bits at the point when you are eating or potentially not planning to eat the correct food choices.

Albeit fat and weight reduction can, in any case, occur, it's more successive and noticeable at the point when the suitable food choices and portions are chosen and planned.

## How Can I Stay Full Longer?

Stay hydrated and eat food enriched in fiber.

## Do I Have to Eat Low Carb?

No, you can eat what you want during your eating window. I suggest eating proportionately and picking on better food choices. Rather than white bread, pick whole grain bread. Rather than white rice, pick brown rice. Rather than anything with high fructose corn syrup, scratch it off; rather than a canned organic product, eat the natural product.

## Should I Exercise in the Fasted State?

It's not mandatorily required to lift heavy weights, but you can do normal day-to-day exercise like yoga, walking, or stretching. Other moderate activities such as running, Swimming or Bicycling are more suitable for those who are already physically trained.

## What If I Am on Medications and Must Eat with My Morning Medications?

In this situation, make sure that your feeding time matches your medication time. In this case, you would need to make your feeding window begin at whatever time you take your meds. I would recommend taking your meds as late as you can in the mornings, but do get authorization of your plan from a medical professional.

## Should I Deliberate This with My Medical Professional Before Beginning the Change?

Truly, you ought to consistently examine diet changes with a clinical expert before you start.

## Why Should You Start Intermittent Fasting?

The main explanation behind beginning this eating regimen plan is to get thinner without changing one's eating routine to an extraordinary level. With this eating routine plan, you are allowed to maintain your body's bulk and stay slender. This is conceivable since, in such a case, that lessens midsection Fat as the eating routine advances. This diet plan requires little change and no convoluted schedules.

## Is Skipping Breakfast Considered Unhealthy for the Body?

This is a myth that a great many people consider as being valid. This generalization should be evaded. Some say that getting up and eating assists the body with getting the energy it needs for the entire day. That may be valid, yet if you are following a solid eating regimen for the remainder of your meals, skipping breakfast ought not to affect your way of life.

## Is It Okay to Take Supplements with an Intermittent Fasting Regimen?

Of course, you can take those supplements but do not forget to check the side effects. Some of them may work in a way that is better than others. For example, Fat-dissolvable vitamins will be more powerful with your meals during eating hours. Pick them over other kinds of supplements.

## Can a Child Fast?

No, it would be an impractical notion for a youngster to fast.

# 30-DAY MEAL PLAN

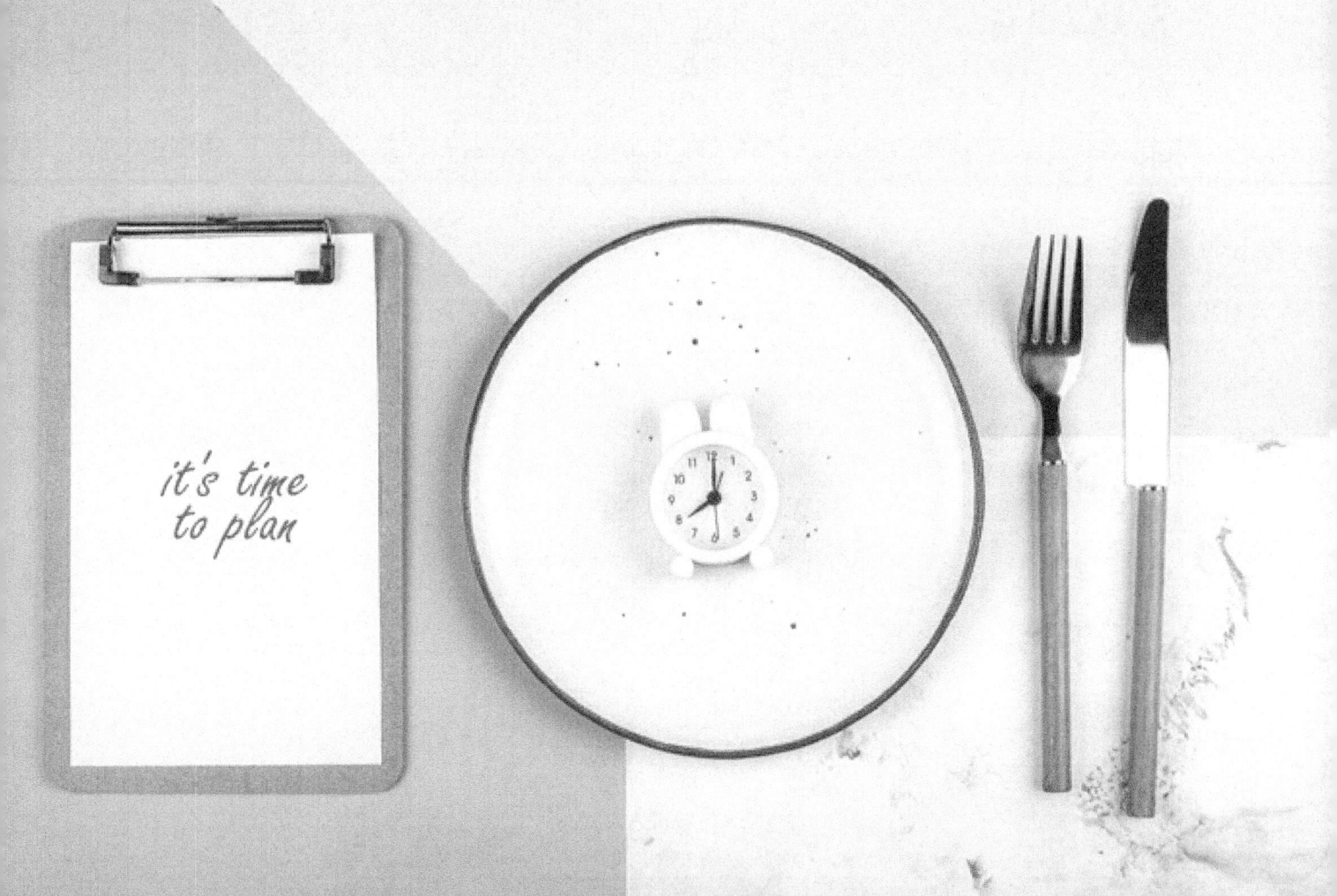

| DAYS | BREAKFAST | LUNCH | DINNER |
|---|---|---|---|
| 1 | Zucchini Omelet | Fragrant Asian Hotpot | Cajun Shrimp |
| 2 | Carrot Breakfast Salad | Salad Skewers | Butternut Squash Risotto |
| 3 | Chocolate Pancakes | Chicken with Kale and Chili Salsa | African Chicken Curry |
| 4 | Coconut Cream with Berries | Tuna and Kale | Mediterranean Lamb |
| 5 | Spinach and Pork with Fried Eggs | Veggie and Beef Salad Bowl | Artichoke Petals Bites |
| 6 | Scrambled Eggs with Halloumi Cheese | Thai Fish Curry | Italian Beef Casserole |
| 7 | Mushroom Omelet | Satisfying Turkey Lettuce Wraps | Lamb Curry |

| DAYS | BREAKFAST | LUNCH | DINNER |
|---|---|---|---|
| 8 | Chili Omelet | Baked Salmon Salad with Creamy Mint Dressing | Garlic Herb Grilled Chicken Breast |
| 9 | Garlic Zucchini Mix | Prawn Arrabbiata | Country Chicken |
| 10 | Breakfast Scramble | Buckwheat Tuna Casserole | Mahi-Mahi Tacos with Avocado and Fresh Cabbage |
| 11 | Seafood Omelet | Artichoke, Chicken and Capers | Beef Cabbage Stew |
| 12 | Smoked Salmon Sandwich | Chicken Merlot with Mushrooms | Healthy Chickpea Burger |
| 13 | Shrimp Deviled Eggs | Turkey with Cauliflower Couscous | Stuffed Beef Loin in Sticky Sauce |
| 14 | Salmon Filled Avocado | Seared Salmon with Braised Broccoli | Camembert Mushrooms |
| 15 | Basil and Cherry Tomato Breakfast | Lamb, Butternut Squash and Date Tagine | Sesame-Crusted Mahi-Mahi |

| DAYS | BREAKFAST | LUNCH | DINNER |
|---|---|---|---|
| 16 | Crustless Broccoli Sun-dried Tomato Quiche | Asian King Prawn Stir Fry with Buckwheat Noodles | Cheesy Broccoli Soup |
| 17 | Oatmeal | Creamy Strawberry & Cherry Smoothie | Fried Whole Tilapia |
| 18 | Coconut Porridge | Cheesy Crockpot Chicken and Vegetables | Yummy Garlic Chicken Livers |
| 19 | Western Omelet | Country Chicken Breasts | Quinoa Protein Bars |
| 20 | Frittata with Fresh Spinach | Mango Chili Chicken Stir Fry | Coated Cauliflower Head |
| 21 | Cauliflower Hash Browns | Turkey with Capers, Tomatoes, and Greens Beans | Healthy Baby Carrots |
| 22 | Mediterranean Vegetable Frittata | White Bean & Veggie Salad | Mediterranean Quinoa with Arugula |
| 23 | Smoked Salmon | Chicken with Orzo Salad | Charred Shrimp, Pesto & Quinoa Bowls |

| DAYS | BREAKFAST | LUNCH | DINNER |
|---|---|---|---|
| 24 | Feta and Spinach Frittata | Mediterranean Chickpea Quinoa Bowl | Greek Cauliflower Rice Bowls with Grilled Chicken |
| 25 | Vegetarian Egg Casserole | Tuna and Spinach Salad | Eggplant & Parmesan |
| 26 | Green Shakshuka | Stuffed Eggplant | Quinoa, Avocado & Chickpea Salad over Mixed Greens |
| 27 | Simple Green Juice | Zoodles Salad | Walnut-Rosemary Crusted Salmon |
| 28 | Banana Walnut Bread with Olive Oil | 15-Minute Couscous with Tuna & Pepperoncini | Spinach & Chicken Skillet Pasta with Parmesan & Lemon |
| 29 | Easy Breakfast Stuffed Mushrooms & Peppers | Greek Chicken and Rice Skillet | Zucchini Lasagna Rolls with Smoked Mozzarella |
| 30 | Easy Pesto Eggs with Tomato and Mozzarella | Harissa Chickpea Stew with Eggplant and Millet | One-Skillet Salmon with Fennel & Sun-Dried Tomato Couscous |

# 150+

## Healthy, Easy & Mouthwatering

# Recipes

### to Stick to Intermittent Fasting Without Sacrificing the Flavor

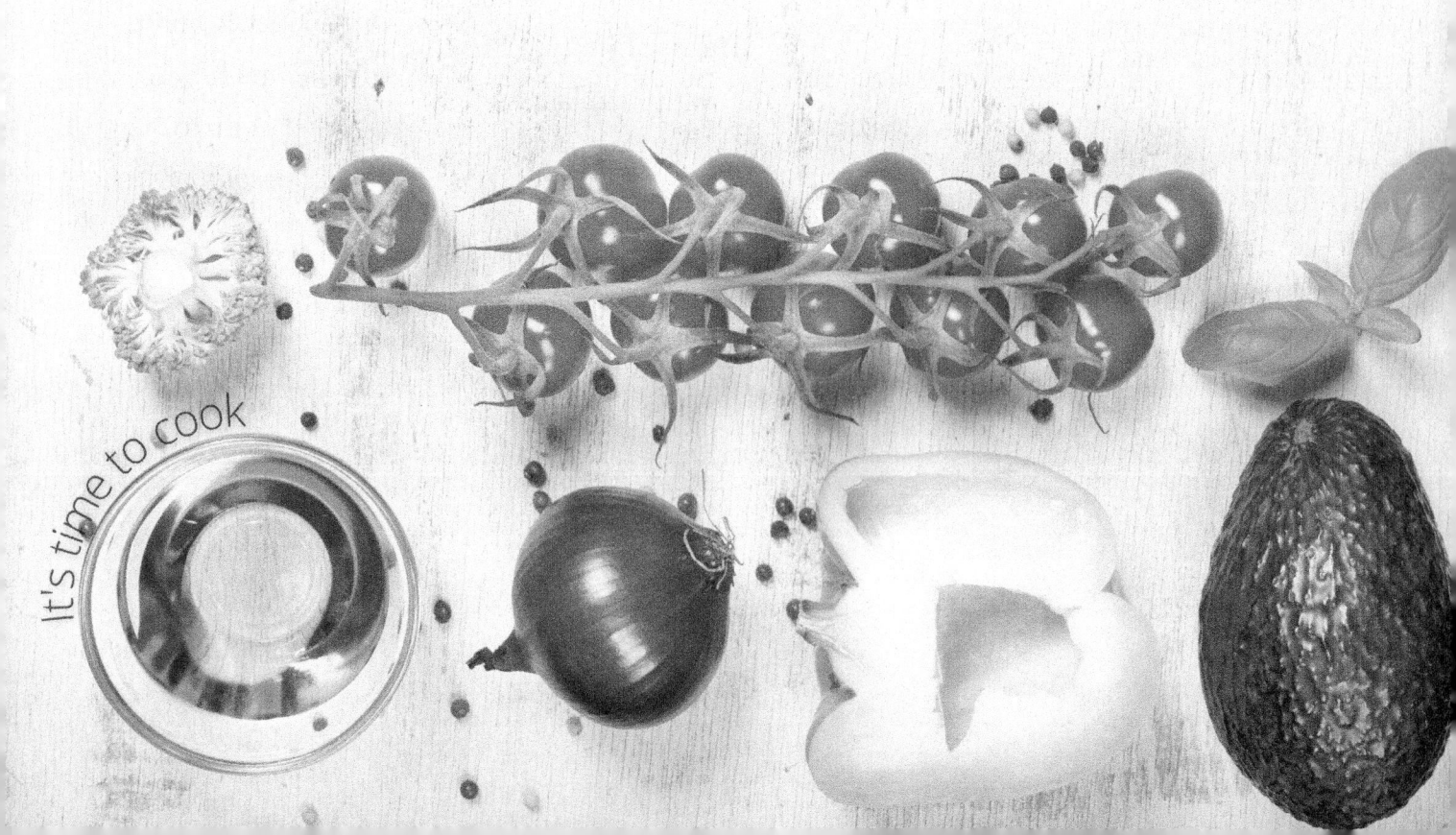

It's time to cook

## Chapter 11: BREAKFAST ................. 67

1. Zucchini Omelet .................................. 67
2. Basil and Cherry Tomato Breakfast ......... 67
3. Carrot Breakfast Salad .......................... 67
4. Broccoli Sun-Dried Tomato Crustless Quiche ................................................ 67
5. Garlic Zucchini Mix ............................... 68
6. Chocolate Pancakes ............................ 68
7. Breakfast Scramble .............................. 68
8. Oatmeal .............................................. 69
9. Coconut Cream with Berries ................ 69
10. Seafood Omelet .................................. 69
11. Spinach and Pork with Fried Eggs ........ 70
12. Spicy Pumpkin Bread ........................... 70
13. Shrimp Deviled Eggs ............................ 70
14. Scrambled Eggs with Halloumi Cheese ................................................ 71
15. Coconut Porridge ................................. 71
16. Western Omelet ................................... 71
17. Mushroom Omelet ................................ 71
18. Frittata with Fresh Spinach .................... 72
19. Cauliflower Hash Browns ...................... 72
20. Salmon-Filled Avocado ........................ 72
21. Creamy Strawberry & Cherry Smoothie ............................................. 73
22. Chili Omelet ......................................... 73
23. Za'atar Olive Oil Fried Eggs ................... 73
24. Mediterranean Vegetable Frittata .......... 73
25. Easy Pesto Eggs with Tomato and Mozzarella .......................................... 74
26. Turkish Scrambled Eggs with Tomatoes ............................................. 74
27. Homemade Granola with Olive Oil and Tahini ......................................... 75
28. Challah Bread ...................................... 75
29. Smoked Salmon ................................... 75
30. Green Shakshuka ................................. 76
31. Jerusalem Bagel ................................... 76
32. Raspberry Clafoutis .............................. 77
33. Shakshuka ........................................... 77
34. Easy Sheets Pan Baked Eggs and Veggies ............................................... 77
35. Simple Green Juice ............................... 78
36. Tahini Banana Date Shakes .................. 78
37. Feta and Spinach Frittata ...................... 78
38. Vegetarian Egg Casserole .................... 79
39. 5-Minute Pumpkin Greek Yogurt Parfait ................................................. 79
40. Banana Walnut Bread with Olive Oil ...... 79
41. Mediterranean Breakfast Egg Muffins .... 80
42. Mediterranean-Style Breakfast Toast .... 80
43. Summer Fruit Compote ........................ 80
44. Zucchini Crustless Quiche .................... 81
45. Easy Breakfast Stuffed Mushrooms & Peppers ............................................... 81
46. Loaded Mediterranean Omelet ............. 82
47. Kuku Sabzi: Baked Persian Herb Omelet ................................................ 82

## Chapter 12: LUNCH ........................ 83

48. Baked Salmon Salad with Mint Dressing ...................................... 83
49. Lamb, Butternut Squash, and Date Tagine ......................................... 83
50. Fragrant Asian Hotpot ........................... 84
51. King Prawn Stir Fry with Buckwheat Noodles ............................................... 84
52. Prawn Arrabbiata .................................. 85
53. Salad Skewers ..................................... 85
54. Chicken with Kale and Chili Sauce ........ 85
55. Buckwheat Tuna Casserole .................. 86
56. Cheesy Crockpot Chicken and Vegetables .......................................... 86
57. Artichoke, Chicken, and Capers with Buckwheat ........................................... 86

58. Chicken Merlot with Mushrooms ............ 87
59. Country Chicken Breasts ......................... 87
60. Tuna and Kale ........................................... 88
61. Turkey with Cauliflower Couscous .......... 88
62. Chicken & Mango Stir Fry ........................ 88
63. Beef and Veggie Salad Bowl .................... 89
64. Turkey with Capers, Tomatoes, and Greens Beans .............................................. 89
65. Thai Fish Curry .......................................... 89
66. Seared Salmon with Braised Broccoli ..... 89
67. Satisfying Turkey Lettuce Wraps ............. 90
68. White Bean & Veggie Salad ..................... 90
69. Greek Meatball Mezze Bowls .................. 90
70. Mediterranean Chickpea Quinoa Bowl ........................................................... 91
71. Tomato, Cucumber & White-Bean Salad with Basil Vinaigrette ...................... 91
72. Tuna and Spinach Salad ........................... 91
73. Mozzarella, Basil, and Zucchini Frittata ...................................................... 92
74. Spinach & Egg Scramble with Raspberries ............................................... 92
75. Chicken with Orzo Salad ......................... 92
76. Mason Jar Power Salad with Chickpeas & Tuna ..................................... 93
77. Creamy Pesto Chicken Salad with Greens ...................................................... 93
78. Chicken Quinoa Bowl .............................. 93
79. Greek Chicken & Cucumber Pita with Yogurt Sauce ........................................... 94
80. Harissa Chickpea Stew with Eggplant and Millet .................................. 94
81. Grilled Lemon-Herb Chicken & Avocado Salad .......................................... 94
82. Minute Heirloom Tomato and Cucumber Toast ....................................... 95
83. Greek Chicken and Rice Skillet ............... 95
84. Mini Chicken Shawarma ......................... 96
85. 15-Minute Couscous with Tuna & Pepperoncini ........................................... 96

86. Pesto Quinoa Bowls with Roasted Veggies and Labneh .............................. 97
87. Greek Yogurt Chicken Salad with Stuffed Peppers ....................................... 97
88. Chicken Skewers with Tzatziki Sauce ..... 97
89. "Zoodles Salad" ......................................... 98
90. Mediterranean Quinoa Bowls ................. 98
91. Greek Lemon Chicken Soup ................... 98
92. Stuffed Eggplant ....................................... 99

### Chapter 13: DINNER .......................... 100

93. Garlic and Herb Grilled Chicken Breast ...................................................... 100
94. Cajun Shrimp ........................................... 100
95. Sesame-Crusted Mahi-Mahi .................. 100
96. Country Chicken .................................... 101
97. Mahi-Mahi Tacos with Avocado and Fresh Cabbage ....................................... 101
98. Butternut Squash Risotto ...................... 101
99. Cheesy Broccoli Soup ............................ 102
100. Beef Cabbage Stew ................................ 102
101. Fried Whole Tilapia ................................ 102
102. African Chicken Curry ........................... 103
103. Yummy Garlic Chicken Livers ............... 103
104. Healthy Chickpea Burger ...................... 104
105. Quinoa Protein Bars ............................... 104
106. Mediterranean Lamb .............................. 104
107. Coated Cauliflower Head ...................... 105
108. Artichoke Petals Bites ............................ 105
109. Stuffed Beef Loin in Sticky Sauce ......... 105
110. Italian Beef Casserole ............................ 106
111. Camembert Mushrooms ....................... 106
112. Lamb Curry ............................................. 106
113. Healthy Baby Carrots ............................. 106
114. Portobello Mushroom Pizzas with Arugula Salad ....................................... 107
115. Mediterranean Quinoa with Arugula .... 107

| | |
|---|---|
| 116. Walnut-Rosemary Crusted Salmon........107 | 137. Chicken with Tomato-Balsamic Pan Sauce................................................116 |
| 117. Cheesy Artichoke & Spinach Spaghetti Squash................................108 | 138. Healthy Lemon Bars.........................116 |
| 118. Mediterranean Stuffed Chicken Breasts..............................................108 | 139. Roasted Pistachio-Crusted Salmon with Broccoli..................................117 |
| 119. Charred Shrimp, Pesto & Quinoa Bowls.................................................109 | **Chapter 14: SNACKS**.....................................118 |
| 120. Sheet-Pan Salmon with Sweet Potatoes & Broccoli..........................109 | 140. Everything-Bagel Crispy Chickpeas......118 |
| 121. Mediterranean Ravioli with Artichokes & Olives............................109 | 141. Kale Chips.........................................118 |
| 122. Slow-Cooker Mediterranean Stew..........110 | 142. Peanut Butter Energy Balls..............118 |
| 123. Greek Cauliflower Rice Bowls with Grilled Chicken..................................110 | 143. Avocado Hummus............................119 |
| 124. Prosciutto Pizza with Corn & Arugula......110 | 144. Fig & Honey Yogurt..........................119 |
| 125. Vegan Mediterranean Lentil Soup..........111 | 145. Cheesy Vegan Brussels Sprout Chips......119 |
| 126. Eggplant & Parmesan.........................111 | 146. Cinnamon-Sugar Roasted Chickpeas..119 |
| 127. B.B.Q. Shrimp with Garlicky Kale & Parmesan-Herb Couscous...............112 | 147. Carrot Cake Energy Bites..................119 |
| 128. Shakshuka with Spinach, Chard & Feta......................................112 | 148. Cucumber Hummus Sandwiches..........120 |
| 129. One-Skillet Salmon with Fennel & Sun-Dried Tomato Couscous...............113 | 149. White Bean & Avocado Toast............120 |
| 130. Spinach & Chicken Skillet Pasta with Parmesan & Lemon..........................113 | 150. Tomato-Basil Skewers......................120 |
| 131. Quinoa, Avocado & Chickpea Salad over Mixed Greens............................113 | 151. Garlic Hummus.................................120 |
| 132. Sheet-Pan Mediterranean Chicken, Brussels Sprouts & Gnocchi..............114 | 152. Savory Date & Pistachio Bites..........121 |
| 133. Caprese Stuffed Portobello Mushrooms......................................114 | 153. Roasted Buffalo Chickpeas...............121 |
| 134. Sweet & Spicy Roasted Salmon with Wild Rice Pilaf...................................114 | 154. Pistachio & Peach Toast....................121 |
| 135. Zucchini Lasagna Rolls with Smoked Mozzarella.........................................115 | 155. Grilled Flatbread with Burrata Cheese..............................................121 |
| 136. Herby Mediterranean Tilapia with Wilted Greens & Mushrooms...............115 | 156. Baked Beet Chips..............................122 |
| | 157. Smoked Salmon and Avocado Summer Rolls....................................122 |
| | 158. Blueberry Coconut Energy Bites............122 |
| | 159. Izy Hossack's Falafel Smash..............123 |
| | 160. Roasted Pumpkin Seeds....................123 |
| | 161. Rainbow Heirloom Tomato Bruschetta.........................................123 |
| | **RECIPES INDEX**..........................**124** |

# CHAPTER 11

# Breakfast

## 1. Zucchini Omelet

**Preparation time:** 4 minutes
**Cooking time:** 3 hours and 30 minutes
**Servings:** 2
**Ingredients:**

- 1½ cups red onion, chopped
- 1 tbsp. olive oil
- 2 garlic cloves, minced
- 2 tsp. fresh basil, chopped
- 6 eggs, whisked
- A pinch of sea salt
- A pinch of black pepper
- 8 cups zucchini, sliced
- 6 oz. fresh tomatoes, peeled, crushed

**Directions:**

1. In a bowl, mix all the ingredients except the oil and the basil.
2. Grease the slow cooker with the oil, spread the omelet mix in the bowl, cover, and cook on low for 3 hours and 30 minutes.
3. Divide the omelet between plates, sprinkle the basil on top, and serve for breakfast.

**Nutrition values per serving:**
Calories: 468Kcal | Protein: 26.5g | Fat: 21.5g | Carbs: 50.1g

## 2. Basil and Cherry Tomato Breakfast

**Preparation time:** 4 minutes
**Cooking time:** 4 hours
**Servings:** 4
**Ingredients:**

- 1 tbsp. olive oil
- 2 yellow onions, chopped
- 2 pounds cherry tomatoes, halved
- 3 tbsp. tomato puree
- 2 garlic cloves, minced
- A pinch of sea salt and black pepper
- 1 bunch basil, chopped

**Directions:**

1. Grease the slow cooker with the oil, add all the ingredients, cover, and cook on high for 4 hours.
2. Stir the mixture, divide it into bowls and serve for breakfast.

**Nutrition values per serving:**
Calories: 100Kcal | Protein: 2.9g | Fat: 4g | Carbs: 15.5g

## 3. Carrot Breakfast Salad

**Preparation time:** 5 minutes
**Cooking time:** 4 hours
**Servings:** 4
**Ingredients:**

- 2 tbsp. olive oil
- 2 pounds baby carrots, peeled and halved
- 3 garlic cloves, minced
- 2 yellow onions, chopped
- ½ cup vegetable stock
- 1/3 cup tomatoes, crushed
- A pinch of salt and black pepper

**Directions:**

1. In your slow cooker, combine all the ingredients, cover, and cook on high for 4 hours.
2. Divide into bowls and serve for breakfast.

**Nutrition values per serving:**
Calories: 169Kcal | Protein: 2.4g | Fat: 7.4g | Carbs: 25.5g

## 4. Broccoli Sun-Dried Tomato Crustless Quiche

**Preparation time:** 4 minutes
**Servings:** 2
**Cooking time:** 3 hours and 30 minutes
**Ingredients:**

- 12.3 oz. box extra-firm tofu drained and dried - 1 ½ cup broccoli, chopped
- 2 tsp. yellow mustard
- 1 tbsp. tahini
- 1 tbsp. cornstarch
- ½ tsp. turmeric

- ¼ cup old-fashioned oats
- ½–1 tsp. salt
- 3–4 dashes of Tabasco sauce
- ½ cup artichoke hearts, chopped
- 2/3 cup tomatoes, sun-dried, soaked in hot water
- 1/8 cup vegetable broth

**Directions:**
1. Preheat your oven to 375°F.
2. Prepare a 9" pie plate or springform pan with parchment paper or cooking spray.
3. Put all leeks and broccoli on a cookie sheet and drizzle with vegetable broth, salt, and pepper Bake for about 20–30 min.
4. In the meantime, add the tofu, garlic, nutritional yeast, lemon juice, mustard, tahini, cornstarch, oats, turmeric, salt, and a few dashes of Tabasco in a food processor. When the mixture is smooth, taste for heat and add more Tabasco as needed. Place cooked vegetables with artichoke hearts and tomatoes in a large bowl. With a spatula, scrape in tofu mixture from the processor Mix carefully so all of the vegetables are well distributed. If the mixture seems too dry, add a little vegetable broth or water.
5. Add mixture to pie plate muffin tins or springform pan and spread evenly.
6. Bake for about 35 min or until lightly browned. Cool before serving. It is delicious, both warm and chilled!

**Nutrition values per serving:**
Calories: 407Kcal | Protein: 34.1g | Fat: 20.7g | Carbs: 30.3g

## 5. Garlic Zucchini Mix

**Preparation time:** 5 minutes
**Cooking time:** 6 hours
**Servings:** 2
**Ingredients:**
- 4 cups zucchinis, sliced
- 2 tbsp. olive oil
- 1 tsp. Italian seasoning
- A pinch of salt and black pepper
- 1 tsp. garlic powder

**Directions:**
1. In your slow cooker, mix all the ingredients, cover, and cook for 6 hours.
2. Divide into bowls and serve for breakfast.

**Nutrition values per serving:**
Calories: 168Kcal | Protein: 3g | Fat: 15.1g | Carbs: 8.9g

## 6. Chocolate Pancakes

**Preparation time:** 5 minutes
**Cooking time:** 80 minutes
**Servings:** 2
**Ingredients:**
- 1 ¼ cups gluten-free flour of choice
- 1 tbsp. ground flaxseed
- 1 tbsp. baking powder
- ¼ tsp. sea salt
- 3 tbsp. nutritional yeast
- 2 tbsp. unsweetened cocoa powder
- 1 cup unsweetened, unflavored almond milk
- 1 tbsp. vegan mini chocolate chips (optional)
- 1 tsp. vanilla extract
- ¼ tsp. stevia powder or 1 tbsp. pure maple syrup
- 1 tbsp. apple cider vinegar
- ¼ cup unsweetened applesauce

**Directions:**
1. Get a medium bowl and mix all the dry ingredients (flour, baking powder, flaxseed, cocoa powder, yeast, salt, and optional chocolate chips). Whisk until evenly combined.
2. In a separate small bowl, combine wet ingredients except for the applesauce (almond milk, vanilla extract, apple cider vinegar, maple syrup, or stevia powder). Add wet ingredient mixture and applesauce to the dry ingredients and mix by hand until ingredients are just combined. The batter should sit for 10 minutes. It will rise and thicken, possibly doubling in size. Heat an electric griddle or nonstick skillet to medium heat and spray with a small amount of nonstick spray, if desired. Scoop batter into 3-inch rounds. Much like traditional pancakes, bubbles will start to appear. When bubbles begin to burst, flip pancakes and cook for 1–2 minutes. Create 12 pancakes.

**Nutrition values per serving:**
Calories: 505Kcal | Protein: 24.7g | Fat: 9.3g | Carbs: 85.6g

## 7. Breakfast Scramble

**Preparation time:** 5 minutes
**Cooking time:** 60 minutes
**Servings:** 2
**Ingredients:**
- 1 large head cauliflower, cut up
- 1 seeded, diced green bell pepper
- 1 seeded, diced red bell pepper

- 2 cups sliced mushrooms (approximately 8 oz. whole mushrooms)
- 1 peeled, diced red onion
- 3 peeled, minced cloves of garlic
- Sea salt
- 1 ½ tsp. turmeric
- 1–2 tbsp. low-sodium soy sauce
- ¼ cups nutritional yeast (optional)
- ½ tsp. black pepper

**Directions:**
1. Sauté green and red peppers, mushrooms, and onion in a medium saucepan or skillet over medium-high heat until onion is translucent (should be 7–8 min). Add an occasional tbsp. or two of water to the pan to prevent vegetables from sticking.
2. Add cauliflower and cook until florets are tenders. It should be 5–6 minutes.
3. Add pepper, garlic, soy sauce, turmeric, and yeast (if using) to the pan and cook for about 5 minutes.

**Nutrition values per serving:**
Calories: 252Kcal | Protein: 21.3g | Fat: 2.1g | Carbs: 48.7g

## 8. Oatmeal

**Preparation time:** 5 minutes
**Cooking time:** 30 minutes
**Servings:** 4
**Ingredients:**
- 1 cup almond milk, unsweetened
- 1 tbsp. flaxseed, whole
- 1 tbsp. sunflower seeds
- 1 tbsp. chia seeds
- ½ tsp. salt

**Directions:**
1. Dump all the ingredients together into a small pan and bring them to a boil over medium heat.
2. When it comes to a boil, reduce the heat and allow the mix to simmer gently for 2–3 minutes until the mixture is the desired thickness.
3. Drop a pat of butter on the top and enjoy.

**Nutrition values per serving:**
Calories: 151Kcal | Protein: 1.8g | Fat: 15.2g | Carbs: 4g

## 9. Coconut Cream with Berries

**Preparation time:** 5 minutes
**Cooking time:** 30 minutes
**Servings:** 4
**Ingredients:**
- ½ cup coconut cream
- 1 tsp. vanilla extract
- 2 oz. strawberries, fresh

**Directions:**
1. Mix the ingredients well by using a hand mixer or an immersion mixer if one is available.
2. An add a tsp. of coconut oil will increase the amount of fat in this dish.

**Nutrition values per serving:**
Calories: 77Kcal | Protein: 0.8g | Fat: 7.2g | Carbs: 2.9g

## 10. Seafood Omelet

**Preparation time:** 5 minutes
**Cooking time:** 30 minutes
**Servings:** 2
**Ingredients:**
- 5 oz. shrimp, cooked
- 6 eggs
- 2 tbsp. butter
- 2 tbsp. olive oil
- 1 tbsp. chives, fresh or dried
- ½ cup mayonnaise.
- 1 tsp. Cumin, ground
- ¼ tsp. thyme
- 2 garlic, cloves minced
- 1 red chili pepper, diced
- ½ tsp. salt
- 1 tsp. white pepper

**Directions:**
1. Toss the shrimp with the olive oil until it is completely covered, and fry it gently with the cumin, garlic, salt, chili pepper, and pepper for 5 minutes.
2. While the shrimp mix cools, beat the eggs and pours them into the skillet.
3. Let the eggs sit undisturbed while they cook until the edges begin to brown and the center has mostly set firm.
4. Then add the chives and the mayonnaise to the shrimp mixture.
5. Pour the shrimp mixture onto the egg that is frying in the skillet and fold the omelet in half, frying for an additional three minutes on each side

**Nutrition values per serving:**
Calories: 736Kcal | Protein: 34g | Fat: 59.8g | Carbs: 18.6g

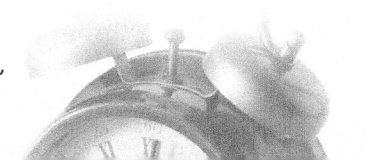

## 11. Spinach and Pork with Fried Eggs

**Preparation time:** 5 minutes
**Cooking time:** 30 minutes
**Servings:** 2.
**Ingredients:**

- 2 cups spinach, baby
- 6 oz. pork loin, smoked, cut into chunks
- 4 eggs
- ½ tsp. salt
- 1 tsp. black pepper
- ¼ cup walnuts, chopped
- ¼ cup cranberries, frozen
- 3 tbsp. butter

**Directions:**

1. Wash, dry, and chop the baby spinach. Fry the spinach in the butter for 5 minutes, stirring continuously.
2. Remove the spinach from the pan and let it drain on a paper towel. Fry the chunks of pork loin in the same skillet for 5 minutes. Remove the pork from the skillet and then put the cooked baby spinach back in, adding the nuts and cranberries. Stir constantly while this is cooking for 5 minutes.
3. Pour the mix into a bowl. Fry the eggs and place 2 on each plate with half of the spinach mixture. Serve with chunks of fried pork loin

**Nutrition values per serving:**
Calories: 598Kcal | Protein: 39.2g | Fat: 47.2g | Carbs: 5.3g

## 12. Spicy Pumpkin Bread

**Preparation time:** 5 minutes
**Cooking time:** 30 minutes
**Servings:** 4
**Ingredients:**

- 1 tbsp. lard
- 14 oz. pumpkin puree
- ¼ cup coconut oil, - 3 eggs
- 1/3 cup pumpkin seeds
- 1/3 cup walnuts, chopped
- 1 tbsp. baking powder
- 2 tbsp. pumpkin pie spice
- ½ cup flaxseed
- 1 tsp. salt
- 1 ¼ cups coconut flour.
- 1 ¼ cups almond flour
- 2 tbsp. psyllium husk powder, ground

**Directions:**

1. Heat oven to 400°F. Use the lard to grease a pan. Add the baking powder, pumpkin pie spice, nuts, psyllium husk powder, flaxseed, both flours, salt, and seeds into a bowl and mix well.
2. Use a separate bowl to cream together the oil, pumpkin puree, and egg. Gently pour this mixture into the dry ingredients, and fold both together until all of the ingredients are well moistened. Spoon this entire mixture into the greased baking pan and bake it for one hour. Allow the bread to cool completely.
3. When the bread is done, beat together the cream and eggs with pepper and salt. Scramble the egg mix in the melted butter for five minutes, stirring constantly, and then mix in the chili powder. Slice off 2 slices of the pumpkin bread and place them in the toaster to toast for 3 minutes. Butter the toasted pumpkin bread and lay each slice on a plate. Top each slice with the kale and the smoked salmon. Place the eggs on top of this and sprinkle with the chives.

**Nutrition values per serving:**
Calories: 666Kcal | Protein: 20.8g | Fat: 53.2g | Carbs: 30.6g

## 13. Shrimp Deviled Eggs

**Preparation time:** 5 minutes
**Cooking time:** 30 minutes
**Servings:** 4
**Ingredients:**

- 1 tsp. chives, chopped
- ¼ cups mayonnaise
- 4 eggs, hard-boiled
- 8 dill sprigs, fresh
- 1 tsp. Tabasco sauce
- 8 shrimp, peeled and deveined, large fully cooked
- ½ tsp. salt
- ½ tsp. white pepper

**Directions:**

1. Carefully peel the chilled hard-boiled eggs and then cut them in half the long way and remove the yolks.
2. Put the yolks into a bowl and use a dinner fork to mash the yolks gently, and then add the Tabasco, salt, and mayonnaise.
3. Mix all of this well, and then carefully spoon the mixture back into the egg whites.
4. Top each egg with one cooked shrimp and a sprig of dill.

NOTE: Shrimp are sold whole or peeled and deveined. You can peel them yourself and remove the vein, but the cost difference to buy them already peeled and deveined (P & D) is very small and worth the price.

**Nutrition values per serving:**

Calories: 173Kcal | Protein: 15.8g | Fat: 10.1g | Carbs: 4.7g

## 14. Scrambled Eggs with Halloumi Cheese

**Preparation time:** 5 minutes
**Cooking time:** 30 minutes
**Servings:** 2
**Ingredients:**

- 4 eggs
- 4 bacon slices
- ½ tsp. salt
- 1 tsp. black pepper
- ¼ tsp. chili powder
- ½ cup black olives, pitted if needed
- ½ cup parsley, fresh, chopped fine
- 2 scallions
- 2 tbsp. olive oil
- 3 oz. halloumi cheese, diced from a block

**Directions:**

1. Chop the bacon and the cheese finely.
2. Fry the bacon and the cheese with the scallions in olive oil for five minutes.
3. While this mixture is frying, beat the eggs well with the parsley, pepper, chili powder, and salt. Dump the egg mix onto the bacon cheese mix in the skillet and scramble all together for 3 minutes while stirring constantly.
4. Add in the olives and cook for 3 more minutes

**Nutrition values per serving:**

Calories: 569Kcal | Protein: 35.5g | Fat: 55.2g | Carbs: 7.3g

## 15. Coconut Porridge

**Preparation time:** 5 minutes
**Cooking time:** 30 minutes
**Servings:** 1
**Ingredients:**

- 1 egg
- ¼ tsp. salt
- 1 tbsp. coconut oil
- 4 tbsp. coconut cream
- ½ tsp. psyllium husk powder, ground
- 1 tbsp. coconut flour

**Directions:**

1. Pour all of the ingredients listed into a pan and mix them together.
2. Cook this mixture over very low heat while constantly stirring until the mixture is the thickness you desire.
3. Serve the porridge with a spoonful of coconut milk or heavy whipping cream and a few frozen or fresh berries if you like.

**Nutrition values per serving:**

Calories: 323Kcal | Protein: 6.9g | Fat: 32.3g | Carbs: 5g

## 16. Western Omelet

**Preparation time:** 5 minutes
**Cooking time:** 30 minutes
**Servings:** 2
**Ingredients:**

- 6 eggs
- 5 oz. smoked deli ham, diced small
- 2 tbsp. butter
- ½ cup green bell pepper, finely chopped
- ¼ cup yellow onion, finely chopped
- 3 oz. shredded sharp cheddar cheese
- 2 tbsp. sour cream
- ½ tbsp. salt
- 1 tsp. black pepper
- 1 tsp. chives, chopped
- ¼ tsp. thyme

**Directions:**

1. Cream together the eggs and the sour cream together until they are fluffy, and season this mix with salt, chives, thyme, and pepper.
2. Sprinkle in just half of the shredded cheese and mix it together well.
3. Cook the peppers, onion, and ham in the melted butter for 5 minutes while stirring often. Dump the egg mixture carefully over the ham mixture in the skillet and cook for an additional 5 minutes just sitting still, do not stir. Sprinkle the remainder of the shredded cheese onto the omelet and carefully fold it in half and fry for 5 more minutes, 2 and one-half minutes per side.

**Nutrition values per serving:**

Calories: 582Kcal | Protein: 39.7g | Fat: 43.9g | Carbs: 7.7g

## 17. Mushroom Omelet

**Preparation time:** 5 minutes
**Cooking time:** 30 minutes
**Servings:** 2

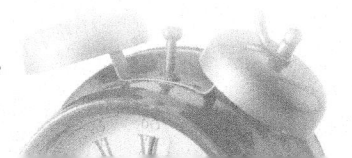

**Ingredients:**

- 3 eggs
- ¼ cup cheddar, shredded
- ½ cup mushrooms
- ¼ cup yellow onion diced fine
- ½ tsp. salt
- ¼ tsp. white pepper
- ½ tsp. rosemary
- 1 tbsp. butter

**Directions:**

1. Break the eggs into a bowl carefully and season them with pepper, salt, and rosemary.
2. Use a fork or a hand mixer to beat the eggs until they are well mixed and slightly frothy.
3. Pour the egg mixture into the melted butter into the pan.
4. Let the omelet cook over medium heat until the half-inch outer edge has begun to look brown and firm and the center half is still slightly raw and wet.
5. Sprinkle the mushrooms, onions, and cheese onto the omelet, staying mostly near the center and away from the cooked edges.
6. Use a spatula to work the edges free of the omelet off the pan and flip one side over onto the other half. Let the omelet cook for 5 more minutes and remove it from the pan.

**Nutrition values per serving:**
Calories: 384Kcal | Protein: 23.2g | Fat: 31.2g | Carbs: 3.5g

## 18. Frittata with Fresh Spinach

**Preparation time:** 5 minutes
**Cooking time:** 30 minutes
**Servings:** 4
**Ingredients:**

- 8 eggs
- 1 cup heavy whipping cream
- 1 tsp. salt
- 1 tsp. black pepper
- ½ tsp. rosemary
- ¼ tsp. thyme
- 5 oz. shredded sharp cheddar cheese, five oz.
- 1 cup spinach, fresh, washed and dried
- 2 tbsp. butter

**Directions:**

1. Heat oven to 350°F. Use 1 tbsp. of lard to grease a 9x9-inch baking pan.
2. Use 1 tbsp. of butter to fry the bacon in a skillet over medium heat. When the bacon is crispy place the cleaned spinach in the skillet, and cook it until the spinach wilts.
3. The bacon will break into pieces while you are stirring it with the spinach. During the time the bacon is cooking, beat the eggs and the heavy cream together in a small bowl.
4. Pour this mix into the baking pan, then add in the spinach and bacon mix and sprinkle all over the top with the sharp cheddar cheese. Bake for 30 minutes and serve hot.

**Nutrition values per serving:**
Calories: 427Kcal | Protein: 20.9g | Fat: 37.4g | Carbs: 2.7g |

## 19. Cauliflower Hash Browns

**Preparation time:** 5 minutes
**Cooking time:** 30 minutes
**Servings:** 4
**Ingredients:**

- 3 eggs, well beaten
- 4 tbsp. butter
- ½ yellow onion, grated
- 1 tsp. black pepper
- 1 tsp. salt
- 1 cauliflower

**Directions:**

1. Wash and rinse the cauliflower and let drain well and then pat it dry.
2. Grate the raw cauliflower finely using a hand grater or a food processor.
3. Dump the finely grated cauliflower into a bowl and add the salt, pepper, egg, and onion.
4. Mix all of this together very well. Form the grated cauliflower mixture into pancake shapes and fry them in the melted butter for 5 minutes on each side If they do not fry long enough, they will break apart when you flip them or remove them from the pan, so do not try to rush them.

**Nutrition values per serving:**
Calories: 208Kcal | Protein: 8.6g | Fat: 15g | Carbs: 13g

## 20. Salmon-Filled Avocado

**Preparation time:** 5 minutes
**Cooking time:** 50 minutes
**Servings:** 2
**Ingredients:**

- 2 avocados
- 2 tbsp. lemon juice
- 1/2 tsp. salt
- 1 tsp. black pepper

- 1 cup sour cream
- 6 oz. smoked salmon

**Directions:**
1. Gently peel the raw avocados and cut them in half the long way, and then remove the pit.
2. Spoon the sour cream into the holes where the pit was and place the smoked salmon on top of the sour cream.
3. Drizzle on the lemon juice and then season to taste with the salt and the pepper.

**Nutrition values per serving:**
Calories: 762Kcal | Protein: 23.2g | Fat: 67.1g | Carbs: 23.2g

## 21. Creamy Strawberry & Cherry Smoothie

**Preparation time:** 10 minutes
**Cooking time:** 15 minutes
**Servings:** 1
**Ingredients:**
- 3½ oz. strawberries
- 3.5 oz. of frozen pitted cherries
- 1 tbsp. natural yogurt
- 6.5 oz. of unsweetened soya milk

**Directions:**
1. Place the ingredients into a blender, then process until smooth. Serve and enjoy!

**Nutrition values per serving:**
Calories: 557Kcal | Protein: 16.7g | Fat: 22.1g | Carbs: 75.5g

## 22. Chili Omelet

**Preparation time:** 5 minutes
**Cooking time:** 3 hours 30 minutes
**Servings:** 4
**Ingredients:**
- 2 garlic cloves, minced
- 1 tbsp. olive oil
- 1 red bell pepper, chopped
- 1 small yellow onion, chopped
- 1 tsp. chili powder
- 2 tbsp. tomato puree
- ½ tsp. sweet paprika
- A pinch of salt and black pepper
- 1 tbsp. parsley, chopped
- 4 eggs, whisked

**Directions:**
1. In a bowl, mix all the ingredients except the oil and the parsley and whisk them well.
2. Grease the slow cooker with the oil, add the egg mixture, cover, and cook on low for 3 hours and 30 minutes.
3. Divide the omelet between plates, sprinkle the parsley on top, and serve for breakfast.

**Nutrition values per serving:**
Calories: 118Kcal | Protein: 6.4g | Fat: 8.2g | Carbs: 6g

## 23. Za'atar Olive Oil Fried Eggs

**Preparation time:** 1 minute
**Cooking time:** 2 minutes
**Servings:** 1
**Ingredients:**
- 1 large egg
- 1 to 2 tbsp. olive oil
- 1/4 tsp. kosher salt
- 2 tsp. za'atar

**Directions:**
1. Split an egg in a small bowl.
2. Warm olive oil in a nonstick skillet on medium heat. Tilt the skillet to spread olive oil and shimmer it.
3. Slide an egg in this heated oil.
4. Add salt & za'atar & cook for 2-3 minutes till the whites are cooked.
5. Serve immediately with your favorite bread.

**Nutrition values per serving:**
Calories: 192.2kcal | Proteins: 5.7g | Fats: 0.1g | Carbs: 1.6g

## 24. Mediterranean Vegetable Frittata

**Preparation time:** 15 minutes
**Cooking time:** 30 minutes
**Servings:** 8
**Ingredients:**
- 1 small red bell pepper
- 1 small zucchini
- 2 green onions
- 4 oz. broccoli
- Kosher salt & black pepper
- 3 tbsp. olive oil
- 7 large eggs
- ¼ tsp. baking powder optional
- ¼ cup whole milk
- ⅓ cup feta cheese, crumbled

- ⅓ cup finely fresh parsley, chopped
- 1 tsp. fresh thyme

**Directions:**
1. Heat the oven at 450 degrees F and place a sheet in an oven for heating.
2. Mix up the bell peppers, green onion, zucchini, & broccoli along with salt & pepper in a bowl. Add olive oil and toss all the ingredients in the oil well.
3. Remove the pan from the oven carefully and spread all the veggies on that heated pan. Again, place the pan in the oven & cook for almost 15 minutes.
4. Turn the heat off when veggies become soft to 400 degrees F.
5. Mix egg, milk, thyme, parsley, feta, baking powder, salt & pepper in a mixing bowl. Fold them out in roasted veggies.
6. Warm the oil on medium heat till shimmering. Pour eggs in a veggie mixture in the pan and cook for 3 minutes to allow the bottom of the eggs to settle.
7. Transfer the pan back to the heated oven and cook for 10 minutes till the center of the eggs are cooked through & the center of the frittata is firm.
8. Serve it with feta cheese and fresh parsley.

**Nutrition values per serving:**
Calories: 136.3kcal | Proteins: 7.8g | Fats: 10.2g | Carbs: 4.2g

## 25. Easy Pesto Eggs with Tomato and Mozzarella

**Preparation time:** 5 minutes
**Cooking time:** 5 minutes
**Servings:** 2
**Ingredients:**
- ⅓ to ½ cup basil pesto
- 2 eggs
- 2 to 3 oz. fresh mozzarella cheese
- 1 vine ripe tomato
- Red pepper flakes
- 2 pieces of toasted bread

**Directions:**
1. Heat the pesto on low heat till shimmering starts in a nonstick pan.
2. Split the eggs & add them into pesto. Cook for 3 minutes till the egg whites become settle down.
3. Add salt, pepper & red pepper flakes.
4. Put this mixture on your toast and arrange tomato, mozzarella on the toast. Slide the eggs & pesto on top as per your liking.

**Nutrition values per serving:**
Calories: 319kcal | Proteins: 14.3g | Fats: 7.8g | Carbs: 6.6g

## 26. Turkish Scrambled Eggs with Tomatoes

**Preparation time:** 10 minutes
**Cooking time:** 15 minutes
**Servings:** 4
**Ingredients:**
- 2 tbsp. olive oil
- 1 medium yellow onion chopped
- 1 green bell pepper
- Kosher salt
- 2 vine-ripe tomatoes
- 3 tbsp. tomato pastes
- black pepper
- ½ tsp. dried oregano
- 1 tsp. Aleppo pepper
- 4 large eggs
- Red pepper flakes, optional, crushed
- 1 French baguette for serving, thickly sliced (optional)

**Directions:**
1. Heat oil in a nonstick skillet and add onions, salt & pepper.
2. Cook for almost 5 minutes till softened.
3. Add tomatoes and paste along with salt, pepper, Aleppo pepper & oregano.
4. Cook it for few minutes on medium heat.
5. Place the tomato and pepper mixture at one side of the pan and lower down the heat.
6. Add the beaten egg and stir gently after cooking till the eggs become settle down.
7. Finish with adding Aleppo pepper along with crushed red pepper flakes.
8. Serve immediately with slices of bread.

**Nutrition values per serving:**
Calories: 164.7kcal | Proteins: 7.2g | Fats: 11.5g | Carbs: 9.3g

## 27. Homemade Granola with Olive Oil and Tahini

**Preparation time:** 15 minutes
**Cooking time:** 40 minutes
**Servings:** 14
**Ingredients:**

- 2 ½ cups rolled oats
- ¾ cup shelled pistachios
- ¾ cup walnuts
- ½ cup sunflower seed
- 3 tbsp. raw sesame seeds
- 1 cup unsweetened coconut flakes
- ¾ cup honey
- ⅔ cup tahini
- ½ cup olive oil
- 2 tsp. pure vanilla extract
- ½ cup light brown sugar
- ½ tsp. ground cinnamon
- ½ tsp. cardamom
- ½ cup chopped Medjool dates
- ½ cup dry cranberries

**Directions:**

1. Heat an oven at 350 degrees F. Add oats, walnuts, pistachios, sesame seeds, coconut flakes and sunflower seeds in a bowl. Mix the honey, cinnamon, vanilla extract, tahini, olive oil, brown sugar, and cardamom in another large bowl.
2. Pour it over an oat mixture & toss till an oat mixture is well-coated.
3. Spread all the mixture on a sheet pan in a single layer. Bake them in the heated oven, stirring after every 8-10 minutes, till the mixture is golden & well-toasted.
4. Allow the granola to cool down after removing it from the heat completely. Break up into clusters & mix along with dates & cranberries.

**Nutrition values per serving:**
Calories: 392kcal | Proteins: 8.1g | Fats: 1.6g | Carbs: 40.1g

## 28. Challah Bread

**Preparation time:** 30 minutes
**Cooking time:** 25 minutes **Servings:** 20
**Ingredients:**

- 2 ¼ tsp. active dry yeast
- 1 cup warm water
- 7 large egg yolks
- 4 cups all-purpose flour
- ¼ cup sugar
- 1 tsp. salt
- 6 tbsp. early harvest olive oil
- 2-3 tbsp. toasted sesame seeds

**Directions:**

1. Mix yeast along with warm water & sugar in a small bowl. Mix them to dissolve yeast for 10 minutes till a foamy yeast layer forms.
2. Mix flour, sugar, salt, oil, & egg yolks in a bowl. Add yeast into this mixture. Mix it well till the dough become hard by using a wooden spoon. Transfer the dough to a floured surface to make it knead and sticky, soft & smooth.
3. Put the dough in an oily bowl and cover it with a kitchen cloth. Kept it warm till the dough rises. Punch the dough down and turn it back to a light flour work surface. Divide the dough into 3 equal pieces. Roll every piece having 16-18 inches long rope & braid the 3 ropes like your hair. Squeeze out both ends to complete the braid. Put the braided loaf on a baking sheet along with parchment paper. Cover it and return to a warm spot for almost more 45 minutes. Allow it to rise again. Heat the oven to 350 degrees F. Sprinkle the sesame seeds after brushing the loaf with egg whites. Bake them out in an oven for 25 minutes till golden brown. Let the challah bread cool down before serving.

**Nutrition values per serving:**
Calories: 124kcal | Proteins: 3.9g | Fats: 6.5g | Carbs: 22.2g

## 29. Smoked Salmon

**Preparation time:** 15 minutes
**Cooking time:** 30 minutes
**Servings:** 6
**Ingredients:**

- 4 soft boiled eggs
- Kosher salt
- Red pepper flakes
- 12 oz. smoked salmon
- 4 oz. cream cheese
- 3 oz. feta cheese
- 1 English cucumber
- 1 bell pepper
- 1 vine-ripe tomato
- 5 radishes

- ¼ cup assorted olives
- ⅓ cup marinated artichoke hearts
- 1 small red onion
- 1 lemon

**Directions:**
1. Bring a saucepan of water and boil eggs on medium heat.
2. Cook for 6 minutes, and when eggs become ready, transfer them to a cooling bowl.
3. Set them aside for 2 minutes. Peel the eggs and cut them into halves. Add salt, red pepper, Aleppo pepper to it.
4. Put a small bowl of labneh to combine the salmon platter. Put feta cheese in another corner of the platter. Arrange the cucumbers, salmon, bell peppers, radish, olives, onions, artichoke, tomatoes & lemon wedges around the cheese. Spray red pepper flakes more on it.
5. Serve it with pita chips, wedges, crackers, and crostini.

**Nutrition values per serving:**
Calories: 197.9kcal | Proteins: 20.3g | Fats: 2.8g | Carbs: 9.6g

## 30. Green Shakshuka

**Preparation time:** 10 minutes
**Cooking time:** 30 minutes
**Servings:** 4
**Ingredients:**
- ¼ cup olive oil
- 3 garlic cloves
- 8 oz. brussels sprouts
- Kosher salt
- ½ large red onion, finely chopped
- 1 large bunch kale (8 oz.)
- 2 cups baby spinach
- 1 tsp. Aleppo pepper
- 1 tsp. coriander
- ¾ tsp. cumin
- Juice of ½ lemon
- 4 large eggs
- 1 green onion
- Fresh parsley for garnish
- Crumbled feta for garnish

**Directions:**
1. Heat the olive oil on medium heat and add Brussel sprouts. Spray with a pinch of salt and cook for 6 minutes till they become soft.
2. Lower down the heat to low. Add garlic and onions into it and mix them for 4 minutes till softened.
3. Add the kale & toss for 5 minutes till it wilts a little. Add the spinach and toss to mix it up well. Add salt more into it as per your requirement and taste.
4. Add all the spices & toss to combine along with ½ cup of water. Convert the heat to medium-low. Cover it and let it cook for 10 minutes till the kale has become completely wilted. Stir it in lemon juice. Split an egg after making 4 wells by using a spoon and season them with salt. Cover them and cook in a pan for 4 minutes till the eggs have become settled. Remove them from the heat. Add another sprinkle of olive oil if you like. Garnish it with parsley, fresh green onions, and some creamy feta.

**Nutrition values per serving:**
Calories: 229.6kcal | Proteins: 9g | Fats: 18.2g | Carbs: 9.8g

## 31. Jerusalem Bagel

**Preparation time:** 30 minutes
**Cooking time:** 15 minutes
**Servings:** 6
**Ingredients:**
- 4 ½ cup all-purpose flour
- 2 tbsp. sugar
- 2 tsp. salt
- 1 ½ cups whole milk
- 1 tbsp. active dry yeast
- 1 tsp. baking powder
- Olive oil

For sesame coating
- 1 cup sesame seeds
- 1 to 2 tbsp. honey

**Directions:**
1. Place the flour, milk, yeast, sugar, salt, and baking powder in the bowl. Mix on medium speed till the dough comes together and forms a soft and pliable ball.
2. Allow the dough to rise.
3. Mix the sesame seeds, water, and honey in a baking bowl. Work on it with a wet mixture till become coating of sesame becomes to prepare for dough sickness.
4. Divide the dough into 6 equal parts and heat the oven to 450 degrees F.

5. Take each dough ring and dip it in the sesame mixture after setting it on a large baking sheet. Repeat it with all the remaining rings.
6. Put the baking sheet in the heated oven for 20 minutes till the bagels cook and turn into golden color.

**Nutrition values per serving:**
Calories: 396.5kcal | Proteins: 11.9g | Fats: 3g | Carbs: 78.9g

## 32. Raspberry Clafoutis

**Preparation time:** 15 minutes
**Cooking time:** 35 minutes
**Servings:** 6
**Ingredients:**
- Unsalted butter
- 3 cups (350g) raspberries
- ½ cup plus 1 tbsp. granulated sugar
- 1 tsp. dried lavender buds, (optional)
- ½ cup whole milk
- ½ cup crème fraiche (optional)
- 4 large eggs
- Pinch salt
- ⅓ cup all-purpose flour (43g)
- Confectioners' sugar for serving

**Directions:**
1. Heat the oven to 375 degrees F. mix the raspberries and sugar in a bowl. Let them sit and prepare other ingredients.
2. Combine the remaining ½ cup sugar along with the lavender in a blender. Process them till the lavender become ground, almost for 2 minutes. Pour the milk, salt, crème Fraiche, eggs, and manage to combine. Add flour & pulse to combine.
3. Set the sugared berries in a prepared baking dish & pour the egg mixture on them. Bake till the cake is golden & the center springs back for about 35 minutes.
4. Transfer the baking dish into a wire rack to cook for almost 15 minutes before serving.

**Nutrition values per serving:**
Calories: 135kcal | Proteins: 5.8g | Fats: 3.9g | Carbs: 33.5g

## 33. Shakshuka

**Preparation time:** 10 minutes
**Cooking time:** 30 minutes
**Servings:** 6
**Ingredients:**
- Olive oil
- 1 large chopped yellow onion
- 2 chopped green peppers
- 2 cloves garlic
- 1 tsp. ground coriander
- 1 tsp. sweet paprika
- 1/2 tsp. ground cumin
- Red pepper flakes pinch (optional)
- Salt and pepper
- 6 chopped vine-ripe tomatoes
- 1/2 cup tomato sauce
- 6 large eggs
- 1/4 cup fresh parsley leaves
- 1/4 cup chopped fresh mint leaves

**Directions:**
1. Heat olive oil in a pan. Add onions, green peppers, spices, pinch salt, garlic, and pepper. Cook till the vegetables have become softened, around 5 minutes.
2. Add tomatoes & tomato sauce. Cover it and let simmer it for around 15 minutes. Uncover it and cook to allow the mixture to reduce & thicken. Taste & adjust seasoning to your liking.
3. Mae 6 wells by using a wooden spoon in the tomato mixture. Gently split eggs in each well. Reduce the heat. Cover the pan and cook till the egg whites are set.
4. Uncover them and add fresh parsley & mint. Serve them immediately with challah bread and pita.

**Nutrition values per serving:**
Calories: 154kcal | Proteins: 9g | Fats: 7.8g | Carbs: 14.1g

## 34. Easy Sheets Pan Baked Eggs and Veggies

**Preparation time:** 10 minutes
**Cooking time:** 15 minutes
**Servings:** 6
**Ingredients:**
- 1 green bell pepper, cored and thinly sliced
- 1 orange bell pepper, cored and thinly sliced
- 1 red bell pepper, cored and thinly sliced
- 1 medium red onion, halved, then thinly sliced
- Salt & black pepper
- Spices of your choice
- Olive oil

- 6 large eggs
- Chopped fresh parsley
- 1 Roma tomato, diced
- Crumbled feta (optional)

**Directions:**
1. Heat an oven to 400 degrees F. put sliced bell peppers in a bow.
2. Add red onions, salt, pepper, cumin, Aleppo pepper, za'atar and olive oil for tossing to coat.
3. Transfer the onion & pepper into a sheet pan. Spread them in a single layer. Bake them in the heated oven for 15 minutes.
4. Remove pan from oven and make 6 holes in the roasted veggies.
5. Split eggs in each hole and place the pan again into the oven. Bake them till the egg whites become settle down.
6. Remove them from the oven and sprinkle feta, tomatoes, and parsley as per your liking.

**Nutrition values per serving:**
Calories: 111kcal | Proteins: 6.9g | Fats: 7.3g | Carbs: 4.5g

## 35. Simple Green Juice

**Preparation time:** 15 minutes
**Cooking time:** 15 minutes
**Servings:** 2
**Ingredients:**
- 1 bunch kale (about 5 oz.)
- 1-inch piece fresh ginger, peeled
- 1 granny smith apple
- 5 celery stalks, ends trimmed
- ½ large English cucumber
- Fresh parsley (about 1 oz.)

**Directions:**
1. Wash out and prepare the veggies. Pour the green juice into glasses and enjoy them.
2. Use a blender for the thickening of juice. Pour out the juice by using the back of a spoon and remove the pulp from the liquid. Serve and enjoy immediately after pouring green stained juice.

**Nutrition values per serving:**
Calories: 92kcal | Proteins: 2.8g | Fats: 0.8g | Carbs: 21g

## 36. Tahini Banana Date Shakes

**Preparation time:** 5 minutes
**Cooking time:** 5 minutes
**Servings:** 3

**Ingredients:**
- 2 frozen bananas
- 4 pitted Medjool dates
- 1/4 cup tahini
- 1/4 cup crushed ice
- 1 1/2 cups unsweetened almond milk
- Pinch ground cinnamon

**Directions:**
1. Put the sliced frozen bananas in a blender. Add all the ingredients and run the blender till creamy shake become achieved.
2. Transfer the banana date shakes into serving cups and add more cinnamon on the top.

**Nutrition values per serving:**
Calories: 225kcal | Proteins: 3.7g | Fats: 12.6g | Carbs: 26.6g

## 37. Feta and Spinach Frittata

**Preparation time:** 10 minutes
**Cooking time:** 12 minutes
**Servings:** 8
**Ingredients:**
- 8 eggs
- 1/4 cup milk
- 1 tsp. dried oregano
- 1/2 tsp. dill weed
- 1/2 tsp. black pepper
- 1/2 tsp. paprika
- 1/4 tsp. baking powder (optional)
- Pinch salt
- 6 oz. frozen spinach, chopped
- 1/2 cup yellow onion, finely chopped
- 1 cup fresh parsley, chopped
- 3 tbsp. fresh mint leaves, chopped
- 3 garlic cloves, minced
- 3 to 4 oz. crumbled feta cheese
- olive oil

**Directions:**
1. Heat oven to 375 degrees F. Mix eggs, salt, and baking powder in a bowl. Add spinach and remaining ingredients into the egg mixture. Mix them well.
2. Heat olive oil in a skillet and pour egg mixture into it. Give the skillet a shake to allow the egg mixture to spread out.
3. Cook on medium heat for 4 minutes and transfer to the heated oven to finish cooking.

**Nutrition values per serving:**

Calories: 152kcal | Proteins: 9.8g | Fats: 10.7g | Carbs: 4.9g

## 38. Vegetarian Egg Casserole

**Preparation time:** 15 minutes
**Cooking time:** 35 minutes
**Servings:** 12
**Ingredients:**

- 7 to 8 large eggs
- 1 1/2 cups milk
- 1/2 tsp. baking powder
- Kosher salt & black pepper
- 1 tsp. dry oregano
- 1 tsp. sweet paprika
- 1/4 tsp. nutmeg
- 3 slices of bread
- 2 shallots, thinly sliced
- 1 small tomato, diced
- 3 oz. sliced mushrooms (any kind; optional)
- 4 oz. artichoke hearts
- 2 oz. pitted kalamata olives
- 2 to 3 oz. crumbled feta cheese
- 1 oz. fresh parsley, chopped
- Olive oil
- 1 bell pepper

**Directions:**

1. Heat the oven to 375 degrees F. mix together milk, eggs, salt, pepper, spices, and baking powder in a bowl.
2. Add the bread pieces, mushrooms, artichoke hearts, shallots, tomatoes, kalamata olives, feta, and parsley into the egg mixture. Mix till everything is properly combined.
3. Brush the bowl with olive oil and transfer the egg and veggie mixture into it. Spread them evenly and put egg casserole at the middle rack of the heated oven.
4. Bake for almost 45 minutes till the eggs are cooked and look firm. Check it by using a toothpick.
5. Allow it for few minutes for the casserole to settle down before cutting and serving.

**Nutrition values per serving:**

Calories: 126kcal | Proteins: 7g | Fats: 6.3g | Carbs: 11g

## 39. 5-Minute Pumpkin Greek Yogurt Parfait

**Preparation time:** 5 minutes
**Cooking time:** 5 minutes
**Servings:** 6
**Ingredients:**

- 1 15-oz. can pumpkin puree
- 1 1/4 cup Greek yogurt
- 3-4 tbsp. mascarpone cheese
- 1 tsp. vanilla extract
- 2 tbsp. molasses, more for garnish
- 2 1/2 tbsp. brown sugar
- 1 1/2-2 tsp. ground cinnamon
- Pinch of ground nutmeg
- Chopped hazelnuts
- Chocolate chips for garnish

**Directions:**

1. Put the ingredients, pumpkin puree and yogurt, in a bowl except for the nuts and chips. Whisk together by using an electric mixer till a smooth mixture is obtained.
2. Please give it a taste & adjust the flavor to your liking.
3. Transfer the mixture to small mason jars. Cover them and refrigerate them for 30 minutes.
4. Top with molasses, walnuts, chocolate chips during serving.

**Nutrition values per serving:**

Calories: 97kcal | Proteins: 5.4g | Fats: 4.6g | Carbs: 9.1g

## 40. Banana Walnut Bread with Olive Oil

**Preparation time:** 15 minutes
**Cooking time:** 55 minutes
**Servings:** 1
**Ingredients:**

- 1/3 cup private reserve olive oil
- 1/2 cup quality honey
- 2 eggs
- 3 bananas, extra ripe
- 2 tbsp. fat-free plain yogurt
- 1/4 cup fat-free milk
- 1 tsp. baking soda
- 1 tsp. vanilla extract
- 1/2 to 3/4 tsp. ground cardamom
- 1/2 tsp. ground cinnamon

- 1/2 tsp. nutmeg, ground
- 1 1/3 cup all-purpose flour
- 6 dates (about 1/2 cup chopped dates)
- 1/3 cup walnut hearts, chopped

**Directions:**
1. Heat the oven to 325 degrees F. whish the oil and honey in a bowl. Add eggs and mix them well.
2. Add bananas yogurt, cinnamon, vanilla extract, milk, baking soda, cardamom, and nutmeg. Whisk again.
3. Stir the flour by using a spatula and add dates, walnuts to mix it well again.
4. Pour them in an oily pan and shake them gently.
5. Bake them in a heated oven. After 50 minutes, test it by using a toothpick for checking the moistness of crumbs.
6. Remove them from the oven and let them cool for 10 minutes.
7. Slice the bread and enjoy it.

**Nutrition values per serving:**
Calories: 200kcal | Proteins: 2.8g | Fats: 6.9g | Carbs: 33.6g

## 41. Mediterranean Breakfast Egg Muffins

**Preparation time:** 15 minutes
**Cooking time:** 25 minutes
**Servings:** 12
**Ingredients:**
- Olive oil for brushing
- 1 small red bell pepper, chopped (about 3/4 cup)
- 12 cherry tomatoes, halved
- 1 shallot, finely chopped
- 6 to 10 pitted kalamata olives, chopped
- 3 to 4 oz. cooked chicken (113g)
- f1 oz. fresh parsley leaves (28. 34g)
- Handful crumbled feta
- 8 large eggs
- Salt & pepper
- 1/2 tsp. spinach paprika
- 1/4 tsp. ground turmeric (optional)

**Directions:**
1. Put a rack in the center of the oven and heat to 350 degrees F.
2. Brush the muffin cup with olive oil after preparing 12 muffin cups.
3. Divide the peppers, shallots, olives, tomatoes, chicken, parsley, and crumbled feta among the 12 cups.
4. Add eggs, pepper, salt, and spices to a bowl. Mix them well.
5. Pour the egg mixture over every cup, leaving a little room at the top.
6. Place muffin cups on top of a sheet pan. Bake them in the heated oven for 25 minutes or till the egg muffins are set.
7. Let them cool for a few minutes, then run a small butter knife around the edges of every muffin to loosen. Remove it from the pan and serve it.

**Nutrition values per serving:**
Calories: 67kcal | Proteins: 4.6g | Fats: 4.7g | Carbs: 1.2g

## 42. Mediterranean-Style Breakfast Toast

**Preparation time:** 10 minutes
**Cooking time:** 10 minutes
**Servings:** 4
**Ingredients:**
- 4 thick bread slices, whole grain
- 1/2 cup hummus
- Za'atar spice blend
- Handful baby arugula
- 1 cucumber
- 1 to 2 Roma tomatoes
- 2 tbsp. chopped olives
- Crumbled feta cheese

**Directions:**
1. Toast the bread slices according to your choice.
2. Spread hummus on every slice and add a sprinkle of za'atar spice and remaining toppings.

**Nutrition values per serving:**
Calories: 166kcal | Proteins: 6.1g | Fats: 4.2g | Carbs: 29.4g

## 43. Summer Fruit Compote

**Preparation time:** 15 minutes
**Cooking time:** 5 minutes
**Servings:** 8-10
**Ingredients:**
- 1 lb. Peaches
- 1 lb. cherries, pitted and halved
- ground cinnamon 1 tsp.
- 2 cups red wine, like merlot
- 3/4 cup cane sugar

- 1 1/2 cup plain fat-free Greek yogurt
- 1 tsp. vanilla extract
- Honey, to your liking

**Directions:**
1. Put sliced peaches and cherries in a large bowl. Spray with cinnamon and set them aside.
2. Mix wine, sugar in a pan, and heat for 5 minutes until the sugar is completely dissolved.
3. Pour hot wine over fruit and set it aside to cool down.
4. In a small bowl, mix vanilla extract, honey, and yogurt.
5. Serve fruit wine with w syrup and honey yogurt. Enjoy.

**Nutrition values per serving:**
Calories: 167kcal | Proteins: 1g | Fats: 0g | Carbs: 10.9g

## 44. Zucchini Crustless Quiche

**Preparation time:** 10 minutes
**Cooking time:** 35 minutes
**Servings:** 8
**Ingredients:**
- 1 medium tomato, sliced into thin rounds
- olive oil
- 1 sliced into rounds zucchini
- 3 shallots, sliced into rounds
- Kosher salt & pepper
- 1 tsp. Spanish paprika
- 1/2 cup shredded mozzarella (nearly 2 oz.)
- 2 tbsp. grated parmesan (about 0.35 oz.)
- 3 large eggs, beaten
- 2/3 cup skim milk
- 1/4 tsp. baking powder
- 1/2 cup all-purpose flour
- 1/4 cup packed fresh parsley (about 0.2 oz.)

**Directions:**
1. Heat the oven at 350 degrees F.
2. Sprinkle with salt on sliced tomatoes after arranging on a paper towel. Leave them a few times and pat dry.
3. Heat olive oil on medium heat and add zucchini, shallots, salt, pepper, and paprika. Increase the heat and toss them till veggies are tender. Transfer the cooked zucchini and shallots mixture to the bottom of the pie bowl. Add mozzarella and parmesan cheese.
4. Mix eggs, paprika, milk, flour, baking powder, and fresh parsley in a bowl.
5. Pour the egg mixture into a pie bowl with the top of the cheese mixture.
6. Bake for 20 to 30 minutes in a heated oven until the egg mixture is well set in the bowl. Remove them from the oven. Serve them.

**Nutrition values per serving:**
Calories: 145kcal | Proteins: 8.4g | Fats: 5.6g | Carbs: 16g

## 45. Easy Breakfast Stuffed Mushrooms & Peppers

**Preparation time:** 20 minutes
**Cooking time:** 20 minutes
**Servings:** 6
**Ingredients:**
- 3 bell peppers
- Water
- Olive oil
- 6 oz. mushrooms
- 1 cup chopped yellow onion
- 10 to 12 oz. gold potatoes
- Salt & pepper
- 3/4 tsp. Aleppo pepper
- 3/4 tsp. organic coriander
- 3/4 tsp. organic cumin
- 1/2 tsp. organic turmeric
- 3 garlic cloves, chopped
- 1/2 cup cherry tomatoes, chopped or sliced
- 1/2 cup fresh parsley, chopped
- 6 eggs

**Directions:**
1. Heat the oven to 350 degrees F. arrange pepper in a skillet and add water to it. Cover it with foil and bake it in the oven for 15 minutes. Add mushrooms in potato hash and toss them till browned. Remove them fr40m the skillet after seasoning with salt.
2. Turn heat on medium level. Add olive oil in a skillet and add onions and potatoes after shimmering of oil. Season them with salt and pepper. Cook them for 5 minutes till the potatoes become tender.
3. Add mushrooms, parsley, and tomato and stir to combine well. Remove them from heat. Stuff every potato with egg and pepper. Bake them for 20 minutes till the eggs become softened. Serve immediately.

**Nutrition values per serving:**
Calories: 179kcal | Proteins: 9.5g | Fats: 5.1g | Carbs: 15.6g

## 46. Loaded Mediterranean Omelet

**Preparation time:** 2 minutes
**Cooking time:** 2 minutes
**Servings:** 2
**Ingredients:**

- 4 large eggs
- 2 tbsp. fat-free milk
- 1/4 tsp. baking powder (optional)
- 1/2 tsp. Spanish paprika
- 1/4 tsp. ground allspice
- Salt & pepper
- 1 1/2 tsp. Olive oil
- 1 Tzatziki sauce
- Warm pita to serve (optional)

Toppings

- 1/2 cup cherry tomatoes, halved
- 2 tbsp. kalamata olives, pitted and sliced
- 1/4 to 1/3 cup marinated artichoke hearts
- 2 tbsp. fresh parsley, chopped
- 2 tbsp. fresh mint, chopped
- Crumbled feta cheese

**Directions:**

1. Add the eggs, milk, spices, salt, baking powder, and pepper to a bowl. Quickly and energetically whisk to combine.
2. Heat olive oil till shimmering and pour the egg mixture into it. Stir it and push the cooked portions towards the edges by tilting the pan. Continue to cook until no egg is left behind uncooked.
3. Remove the skillet from heat and add some toppings over the omelet. Use the spatula to fold. Add the remainder of the toppings on top. Spray more herbs on it.
4. Slice the omelet and serve them.

**Nutrition values per serving:**
Calories: 168kcal | Proteins: 13.8g | Fats: 10.7g | Carbs: 4g

## 47. Kuku Sabzi: Baked Persian Herb Omelet

**Preparation time:** 20 minutes
**Cooking time:** 20 minutes
**Servings:** 6
**Ingredients:**

- 5 tbsp. olive oil
- 2 cups flat-leaf parsley leaves
- 2 cups cilantro, leaves and tender stems
- 1 cup fresh dill, roughly chopped
- 6 scallions, chopped
- 1 1/2 tsp. baking powder
- 1 tsp. kosher salt
- 3/4 tsp. ground green cardamom
- 3/4 tsp. ground cinnamon
- 1/2 tsp. ground cumin
- 1/4 tsp. ground black pepper
- 6 large eggs
- 1/2 cup walnuts (optional)
- 1/3 cup dried cranberries (optional)

**Directions:**

1. Heat the oven to 375 degrees F.
2. Coat the sides and bottom of the pan with olive oil. Combine the dill, cilantro, parsley, scallions, and olive oil in a food processor. Process till gently ground. Set them aside.
3. Whisk the baking powder, cardamom, cumin, cinnamon, and salt, pepper in a bowl. Whisk till blended. Add remaining eggs and combine them well. Pout in the prepared pan and fold in the herb scallion mixture.
4. Bake in an oven till the egg become firm for 25 minutes.
5. Let them cool for 10 minutes and cut with a knife to loosen the Kuku. Invert into a plate and remove the parchment paper from the bottom side.
6. Re-invert on cutting board and slice them into wedges and serve them at room temperature.

**Nutrition values per serving:**
Calories: 184kcal | Proteins: 7.1g | Fats: 16.7g | Carbs: 5.1g

# CHAPTER 12

# Lunch

## 48. Baked Salmon Salad with Mint Dressing

**Preparation time:** 20 minutes
**Cooking time:** 20 minutes
**Servings:** 1
**Ingredients:**

- 1 salmon fillet
- Mixed salad leaves
- 2 radishes, trimmed and thinly sliced
- 2 oz. young spinach leaves
- 5 cm piece cucumber, cut into chunks
- One small handful of parsley, roughly chopped
- 2 spring onions, trimmed and sliced

For the dressing:

- 1 tbsp. natural yogurt
- 1 tsp. low-fat mayonnaise
- 2 leaves mint, finely chopped
- 1 tbsp. rice vinegar
- Salt and freshly ground black pepper

**Directions:**

1. Firstly, you heat the oven to 200°C (180°C fan/Gas 6).
2. Place the salmon filet on a baking tray and bake for 16–18 minutes until you have just cooked.
3. Remove, and set aside from the oven. The salmon in the salad is equally nice and hot or cold. If your salmon has skin, cook it skin side down and separate the salmon from the skin using a fish slice after it has fully cooked.
4. Mix the mayonnaise, yogurt, rice wine vinegar, mint leaves, and salt and pepper in a small dish and let it stand for at least 5 minutes for aromas to evolve.
5. Place on a serving plate the salad leaves and spinach, and top with the radishes, the cucumber, the spring onions, and the parsley. Flake the cooked salmon over the salad and sprinkle over the dressing.

**Nutrition values per serving:**
Calories: 381Kcal | Protein: 41g | Fat: 14.3g | Carbs: 21g

## 49. Lamb, Butternut Squash, and Date Tagine

**Preparation time:** 15 minutes
**Cooking time:** 40 minutes
**Servings:** 4
**Ingredients:**

- 2 tbsp. olive oil
- 2 cm ginger, grated
- 1 red onion, sliced
- 3 garlic cloves, grated or crushed
- 1 tsp. chili flake (or to taste)
- 1 cinnamon stick
- 2 tsp. cumin seeds
- 2 tsp. ground turmeric
- ½ tsp. salt
- 4 lamb neck fillets, cut into 2cm chunks
- ½ cup Medjool dates, pitted and chopped
- 14 oz. tin chopped tomatoes, plus half a can of water
- 14 oz. tin chickpeas, drained
- 15.5 oz. butternut squash, cut into 1cm cubes
- 2 tsp. fresh coriander (plus extra for garnish)
- 3 cups buckwheat, couscous, flatbreads, or rice to serve

**Directions:**

1. Preheat the oven until 140°C.
2. Sprinkle about 2 tsp. Olive oil in a large oven-proof casserole dish or cast-iron pot. Put the sliced onion and cook on a gentle heat until the onions are softened but not brown, with the lid on for about 5 minutes.
3. Add chili, cumin, cinnamon, and turmeric to the grated garlic and ginger. Remove well and cook the lid off for one more minute. If it gets too dry, add a drop of water.
4. Add pieces of lamb. In the onions and spices, stir well to coat the meat and then add salt, chopped

dates, and tomatoes, plus about half a can of water (100–200ml).
5. Bring the tagine to a boil, then put the lid on and put it for 1 hour and 15 minutes in your preheated oven.
6. Add the chopped butternut squash and drained chickpeas 30 minutes before the end of the cooking time. Stir all together, bring the lid back on and go back to the oven for the remaining 30 minutes of cooking.
7. Remove from the oven when the tagine is finished and stir through the chopped coriander. Serve with couscous, buckwheat, flatbreads, or basmati rice.

NOTE: If you don't own an oven-proof casserole dish or cast-iron casserole, cook the tagine in a regular casserole until it has to go into the oven and then transfer the tagine to a regular lidded casserole dish before placing it in the oven. Add 5 minutes of cooking time to provide enough time to heat the casserole dish.

**Nutrition values per serving:**
Calories: 441Kcal | Protein: 29.7g | Fat: 13.1g | Carbs: 53.9g |

## 50. Fragrant Asian Hotpot

**Preparation time:** 15 minutes
**Cooking time:** 45 minutes
**Servings:** 2
**Ingredients:**

- 1 tsp. tomato purée
- 1-star anise, crushed (or 1/4 tsp. ground anise)
- Small handful parsley, stalks finely chopped
- 1/2 lime juice.
- Small handful coriander, stalks finely chopped
- 500 ml chicken stock, fresh or made with 1 cube
- 1/2 carrot, peeled and cut
- 1/4 cup beansprouts
- 1/4 cup broccoli, cut into small florets
- 1 tbsp. good-quality miso paste
- 3.5 oz. raw tiger prawns
- 1.76 oz. rice noodles that are cooked according to packet instructions
- Cooked water chestnuts, drained
- 3.5 oz. firm tofu, chopped
- Little sushi ginger, chopped

**Directions:**
1. In a large saucepan, put the tomato purée, star anise, parsley stalks, coriander stalks, lime juice, and chicken stock and bring to boil for 10 minutes.
2. Stir in the carrot, broccoli, prawns, tofu, noodles, and water chestnuts, and cook gently until the prawns are cooked. Take it from heat and stir in the ginger sushi and the paste miso.
3. Serve sprinkled with peregrine leaves and coriander.

**Nutrition values per serving:**
Calories: 201Kcal | Protein: 19.8g | Fat: 3.3g | Carbs: 25.5g

## 51. King Prawn Stir Fry with Buckwheat Noodles

**Preparation time:** 10 minutes
**Cooking time:** 20 minutes
**Servings:** 1
**Ingredients:**

- 2.5 oz. shelled raw king prawns, deveined
- 2 tsp. tamaris
- 1.8 oz. soba (buckwheat noodles)
- 2 tsp. extra virgin olive oil
- 1 garlic clove, finely chopped
- 1 bird's eye chili, finely chopped
- 1 tsp. finely chopped fresh ginger
- Celery, trimmed and sliced
- Red onions, sliced
- Green beans, chopped
- 1.76 oz. kale, roughly chopped
- Chicken stock

**Directions:**
1. Heat a frying pan over a high flame, then cook the prawns for 2–3 minutes in 1 tsp. tamari and 1 tsp. oil. Place the prawns onto a tray. Wipe the pan out with paper from the kitchen, as you will be using it again.
2. Cook the noodles for 5–8 minutes in boiling water or as directed on the packet Drain and put away.
3. Meanwhile, over medium-high heat, fry the garlic, chili, and ginger, red onion, celery, beans, and kale in the remaining oil for 2–3 minutes. Add the stock and boil, then cook for one or two minutes until the vegetables are cooked but crunchy.
4. Add the prawns, noodles, and leaves of lovage/celery to the pan, bring back to the boil, then remove and eat.

**Nutrition values per serving:**
Calories: 670Kcal | Protein: 29.7g | Fat: 27.5g | Carbs: 78.1g

## 52. Prawn Arrabbiata

**Preparation time:** 10 minutes
**Cooking time:** 40 minutes   **Servings:** 1
**Ingredients:**

- Raw or cooked prawns (Ideally king prawns)
- 1.5 oz. buckwheat pasta
- 1 tbsp. extra-virgin olive oil

For the arrabbiata sauce:

- Red onion, finely chopped
- 1 garlic clove, finely chopped
- 1.2 oz. celery, finely chopped
- 1 bird's eye chili, finely chopped
- 1 tsp. dried mixed herbs
- 1 tsp. extra-virgin olive oil
- 2 tbsp. white wine (optional)
- 14 oz. tinned chopped tomatoes
- 1 tbsp. chopped parsley

**Directions:**

1. Firstly, you fry the onion, garlic, celery, and chili over medium-low heat and dry herbs in the oil for 1–2 minutes. Switch the flame to medium, then add the wine and cook for 1 minute. Add the tomatoes and leave the sauce to cook for 20–30 minutes over medium-low heat until it has a nice rich consistency. If you feel the sauce becomes too thick, add some water. While the sauce is cooking, boil a pan of water, and cook the pasta as directed by the packet. Drain, toss with the olive oil when cooked to your liking, and keep in the pan until needed.
2. Add the raw prawns to the sauce and cook for another 3–4 minutes until they have turned pink and opaque, then attach the parsley and serve. If you use cooked prawns, add the parsley, bring the sauce to a boil and eat.
3. Add the cooked pasta to the sauce, blend well, and then serve gently.

**Nutrition values per serving:**
Calories: 441Kcal | Protein: 16.3g | Fat: 16.2g | Carbs: 57.1g

## 53. Salad Skewers

**Preparation time:** 10 minutes
**Cooking time:** 0 minutes
**Servings:** 1
**Ingredients:**

- 2 wooden skewers, soaked in water for 30 minutes before use - 8 large black olives
- 8 cherry tomatoes
- 1 yellow pepper, cut into eight squares
- ½ red onion, chopped in half and separated into eight pieces
- 3.5 oz. (about 10cm) cucumber, cut into four slices and halved
- 3.5 oz. feta, cut into eight cubes

For the dressing:

- 1 tbsp. extra virgin olive oil
- 1 tsp. balsamic vinegar - Juice of ½ lemon
- Few leaves basil, finely chopped (or ½ tsp. dried mixed herbs to replace basil and oregano)
- A right amount of salt and freshly ground black pepper - Few leaves oregano, finely chopped
- ½ clove garlic, peeled and crushed

**Directions:**

1. Thread each skewer with ingredients in the following order: olive, tomato, yellow pepper, red onion, cucumber, feta, basil, olive, yellow pepper, red ointment, cucumber, feta.
2. Put all the ingredients of the dressing in a small bowl and blend well together. Pour over the spoils.

**Nutrition values per serving:**
Calories: 1250Kcal | Protein: 70.3g | Fat: 77.5g | Carbs: 83.5g

## 54. Chicken with Kale and Chili Sauce

**Preparation time:** 5 minutes
**Cooking time:** 45 minutes
**Servings:** 1
**Ingredients:**

- 3 oz. buckwheat
- 1 tsp. chopped fresh ginger
- Juice of ½ lemon, divided
- 2 tsp. ground turmeric
- 3 oz. kale, chopped
- 1.3 oz. red onion, sliced
- 4 oz. skinless, boneless chicken breast
- 1 tbsp. extra-virgin olive oil
- 1 tomato - 1 handful parsley
- 1 bird's eye chili, chopped

**Directions:**

1. Start with the salsa: remove the eye out of the tomato and finely chop it, making sure to keep as much of the liquid as you can. Mix it with chili, parsley, and lemon juice. You could add everything to a blender for different results.
2. Heat your oven to 220°F. Marinate the chicken with a little oil, 1 tsp. of ground turmeric, and lemon juice. Let it rest for 5–10 minutes. Heat a

pan over medium heat until it is hot, then add marinated chicken and allow it to cook for a minute on both sides until it is pale gold). Transfer the chicken to the oven. If the pan is not ovenproof, place it in a baking tray and bake for 8–10 minutes or until it is cooked through. Take the chicken out of the oven, cover with foil, and let it rest for 5 minutes before you serve.

3. Meanwhile, in a steamer, steam the kale for about 5 minutes. In a little oil, fry the ginger and red onions until they are soft but not colored, and then add in the cooked kale and fry it for a minute. Cook the buckwheat in accordance with the packet directions with the remaining turmeric. Serve alongside the vegetables, salsa, and chicken.

**Nutrition values per serving:**
Calories: 643Kcal | Protein: 40.6g | Fat: 21.6g | Carbs: 79.7g

## 55. Buckwheat Tuna Casserole

**Preparation time:** 10 minutes
**Cooking time:** 35 minutes
**Servings:** 2
**Ingredients:**

- 2 tbsp. butter
- 10 oz. package buckwheat ramen noodles
- 2 cups boiling water
- 1/3 cup dry red wine
- 3 cups milk
- 2 tbsp. dried parsley
- 2 tsp. turmeric
- ½ tsp. curry powder
- 2 tsp. all-purpose flour
- 2 cups celery, chopped
- 1 cup frozen peas
- 2 cans tuna, drained

**Directions:**

1. Dot butter into your crockpot and grease the pot.
2. Place buckwheat ramen noodles in a large bowl and pour boiling water to cover. Let sit for 5–8 minutes, or until noodles separate when prodded with a fork.
3. In a separate bowl, whisk together red wine, milk, parsley, turmeric, and flour.
4. Fold in celery, peas, and tuna.
5. Drain the ramen and place it into the crockpot, pouring the tuna mixture over top Mix to combine. Cover and cook on Low 7–9 hours, stirring occasionally.

**Nutrition values per serving:**
Calories: 1263Kcal | Protein: 69.7g | Fat: 34.9g | Carbs: 155.4g

## 56. Cheesy Crockpot Chicken and Vegetables

**Preparation time:** 10 minutes
**Cooking time:** 45 minutes
**Servings:** 2
**Ingredients:**

- 1/3 cup ham, diced
- 3 carrots, chopped
- 3 stalks celery, chopped
- 1 small yellow onion, diced
- 2 cups mushrooms, sliced
- 1 cup green beans, chopped
- ¼ cup water
- 4 boneless, skinless chicken breasts, cubed
- 1 cup chicken broth
- 1 cup milk
- 1 tbsp. parsley, chopped
- ¾ tsp. poultry seasoning
- 1 tbsp. all-purpose flour
- 1 cup cheddar cheese, shredded
- ¼ cup parmesan, shredded

**Directions:**

1. In a large bowl, combine ham, carrots, celery, onion, mushrooms, and green beans. Mix and transfer to your crockpot.
2. Layer the chicken on top without mixing.
3. In the bowl, now empty, whisk broth, milk, parsley, poultry seasoning, and flour together until well combined.
4. Fold in the cheddar and Parmesan.
5. Pour the mixture over the chicken. DO NOT STIR.
6. Cover and cook on high 3–4 hours, or low 6–8 hours.

**Nutrition values per serving:**
Calories: 592Kcal | Protein: 50.5g | Fat: 30.2g | Carbs: 30.9g

## 57. Artichoke, Chicken, and Capers with Buckwheat

**Preparation time:** 10 minutes
**Cooking time:** 55 minutes
**Servings:** 4
**Ingredients:**

- 6 boneless, skinless chicken breasts
- 2 cups mushrooms, sliced

- 1 (14 ½ oz.) can diced tomatoes
- 1 (8 or 9 oz.) package frozen artichokes
- 1 cup chicken broth
- ¼ cup dry white wine
- 1 medium yellow onion, diced
- ½ cup Kalamata olives, sliced
- ¼ cup capers, drained
- 3 tbsp. chia seeds
- 3 tsp. curry powder
- 1 tsp. turmeric
- 3/4 tsp. dried lovage
- Salt and pepper to taste
- 3 cups hot cooked buckwheat

**Directions:**
1. Rinse chicken & set aside.
2. In a large bowl, combine mushrooms, tomatoes with juice, frozen artichoke hearts, chicken broth, white wine, onion, olives, and capers.
3. Stir in chia seeds, curry powder, turmeric, lovage, salt, and pepper.
4. Pour half the mixture into your crockpot, add the chicken, and pour the remainder of the sauce over the top.
5. Cover and cook on Low for 7 to 8 hours or on High for 3 ½–4 hours.
6. Serve with hot cooked buckwheat.

**Nutrition values per serving:**
Calories: 606Kcal | Protein: 73.2g | Fat: 18.8g | Carbs: 37.1g

## 58. Chicken Merlot with Mushrooms

**Preparation time:** 10 minutes
**Cooking time:** 40 minutes **Servings:** 4
**Ingredients:**

- 6 boneless, skinless chicken breasts, cubed
- 3 cups mushrooms, sliced
- 1 large red onion, chopped
- 2 garlic cloves, minced
- ¾ cups chicken broth
- 1 (6 oz.) can tomato paste
- ¼ cups Merlot
- 3 tbsp. chia seeds
- 2 tbsp. basil, chopped finely
- 2 tsp. sugar
- Salt and pepper to taste
- 1 (10 oz.) package buckwheat ramen noodles, cooked
- 2 tbsp. parmesan shaved

**Directions:**
1. Rinse chicken; set aside.
2. Add mushrooms, onion, and garlic to the crockpot and mix. Place chicken cubes on top of the vegetables and do not mix. In a large bowl, combine broth, tomato paste, wine, chia seeds, basil, sugar, salt, and pepper Pour over the chicken. Cover and cook on low for 7–8 hours or on high for 3 ½–4 hours.
3. To serve, spoon chicken, mushroom mixture, and sauce over hot cooked buckwheat ramen noodles. Top with shaved Parmesan.

**Nutrition values per serving:**
Calories: 641Kcal | Protein: 69.8g | Fat: 18.2g | Carbs: 45.2g

## 59. Country Chicken Breasts

**Preparation time:** 10 minutes
**Cooking time:** 45 minutes
**Servings:** 4
**Ingredients:**

- 2 medium green apples, diced
- 1 small red onion, finely diced
- 1 small green bell pepper, chopped
- 3 garlic cloves, minced
- 2 tbsp. dried currants
- 1 tbsp. curry powder
- 1 tsp. turmeric
- 1 tsp. ground ginger
- ¼ tsp. chili pepper flakes
- 1 can (14 ½ oz.) diced tomatoes
- 6 skinless, boneless chicken breasts, halved
- ½ cup chicken broth
- 1 cup long-grain white rice
- 1-pound large raw shrimp, shelled and deveined
- Salt and pepper to taste
- Chopped parsley
- 1/3 cup slivered almonds

**Directions:**
1. Rinse chicken, pat dry, and set aside.
2. In a large crockpot, combine apples, onion, bell pepper, garlic, currants, curry powder, turmeric, ginger, and chili pepper flakes. Stir in tomatoes.
3. Arrange chicken, overlapping pieces slightly, on top of tomato mixture.
4. Pour in broth and do not mix or stir.
5. Cover and cook for 6–7 hours on low.
6. Preheat oven to 200°F. Carefully transfer chicken to an oven-safe plate, cover lightly, and keep warm in the oven. Stir rice into the remaining liquid Increase cooker heat setting to

high; cover and cook, stirring once or twice, until rice is almost tender to bite, 30–35 minutes. Stir in shrimp, cover, and cook until shrimp are opaque in center, about 10 more minutes. Meanwhile, toast almonds in a small pan over medium heat until golden brown, 5–8 minutes, stirring occasionally.
7. Set aside. To serve, season the rice mixture to taste with salt and pepper. Mound in a warm serving dish and arrange chicken on top. Sprinkle with parsley and almonds.

**Nutrition values per serving:**
Calories: 475Kcal | Protein: 40.8g | Fat: 7.4g | Carbs: 61.3g

## 60. Tuna and Kale

**Preparation time:** 5 minutes
**Cooking time:** 20 minutes
**Servings:** 4
**Ingredients:**
- 1-pound tuna fillets, boneless, skinless, and cubed
- 2 tbsp. olive oil
- 1 cup kale, torn
- ½ cup cherry tomatoes, cubed
- 1 yellow onion, chopped

**Directions:**
1. Heat up a pan with the oil over medium heat, add the onion and sauté for 5 minutes.
2. Add the tuna and the other ingredients, toss, cook everything for 15 minutes more, divide between plates and serve.

**Nutrition values per serving:**
Calories: 241Kcal | Protein: 35g | Fat: 8.5g | Carbs: 5.2g

## 61. Turkey with Cauliflower Couscous

**Preparation time:** 20 minutes
**Cooking time:** 50 minutes
**Servings:** 1
**Ingredients:**
- 3 oz. turkey
- 2 oz. cauliflower
- 2 oz. red onion
- 1 tsp. fresh ginger
- 1 pepper bird's eye
- 1 garlic clove
- 3 tbsp. extra virgin olive oil
- 2 tsp. turmeric
- 1.3 oz. dried tomatoes
- 0.3 oz. parsley
- Dried sage to taste
- 1 tbsp. capers
- 1/4 fresh lemon juice

**Directions:**
1. Blend the raw cauliflower tops and cook them in a tsp. extra virgin olive oil, garlic, red onion, chili pepper, ginger, and a tsp. turmeric.
2. Leave to flavor on the fire for a minute, then add the chopped sun-dried tomatoes and 5 g of parsley. Season the turkey slice with a tsp. extra virgin olive oil, the dried sage, and cook it in another tsp. extra virgin olive oil. Once ready, season with a tbsp. caper, 1/4 of lemon juice, 5 g of parsley, a tbsp. water and add the cauliflower

**Nutrition values per serving:**
Calories: 580Kcal | Protein: 28.1g | Fat: 47.2g | Carbs: 15.9g

## 62. Chicken & Mango Stir Fry

**Preparation time:** 25 minutes
**Cooking time:** 5 minutes
**Servings:** 4
**Ingredients:**
- ½ tbsp. sesame oil
- 1 tbsp. low-sodium soy sauce
- 1 tbsp. cornstarch
- 1 lb. chicken thighs, skinless, boneless, diced
- ½ tbsp. peanut oil
- 1 tbsp. minced fresh ginger
- 1 red onion, chopped
- 2 cups snow peas
- 1 tbsp. chili garlic sauce
- 1 mango, peeled, chopped
- 1/8 tsp. sea salt
- 1/8 tsp. black pepper

**Directions:**
1. In a large mixing bowl, combine sesame oil, soy sauce, cornstarch, and chicken; let sit for at least 20 minutes.
2. In a large skillet, heat peanut oil and then sauté ginger and onion for about 2 minutes; add snow peas and stir fry for about 1 minute.
3. Add chicken with the marinade and stir fry for about 2 minutes or until chicken is browned. Add chili sauce, mango, salt, and pepper, and continue stir-frying for 1 minute or until chicken is cooked through and mango is tender.
4. Serve the stir fry over cooked brown rice.

**Nutrition values per serving:**
Calories: 354Kcal | Protein: 37g | Fat: 12.4g | Carbs: 24g

Healthy Recipes

## 63. Beef and Veggie Salad Bowl

**Preparation time:** 10 minutes
**Cooking time:** 15 minutes
**Servings:** 2
**Ingredients:**

- 2 tbsp. dry red quinoa
- ½ cups chopped broccoli florets
- 3 oz. cooked lean beef, diced
- 2 cups mixed greens (arugula, baby spinach, romaine lettuce)
- ¼ red bell pepper, chopped
- 1 tsp. red wine vinegar
- 2 tsp. extra virgin olive oil

**Directions:**

1. Follow package directions to cook quinoa.
2. In a large bowl, toss cooked quinoa with broccoli, beef, greens, and bell pepper.
3. In a small bowl, whisk together vinegar and oil and pour over the salad. Serve.

**Nutrition values per serving:**
Calories: 289Kcal | Protein: 20.4g | Fat: 8.4g | Carbs: 33.3g

## 64. Turkey with Capers, Tomatoes, and Greens Beans

**Preparation time:** 15 minutes
**Cooking time:** 20 minutes
**Servings:** 4
**Ingredients:**

- 1 tbsp. extra-virgin olive oil
- 6 oz. turkey
- ¼ cups capers
- ¼ cups diced fresh tomatoes
- Steamed green beans for serving

**Directions:**

1. Heat oil in a pan; add turkey and fry until golden brown and cooked through.
2. Remove the cooked turkey from the pan and transfer to a plate; add capers and tomatoes to the pan and cook until juicy. Spoon the caper mixture over the turkey and serve with steamed green beans.

**Nutrition values per serving:**
Calories: 289Kcal | Protein: 20.4g | Fat: 8.4g | Carbs: 33.3g

## 65. Thai Fish Curry

**Preparation time:** 5 minutes
**Cooking time:** 10 minutes
**Servings:** 2
**Ingredients:**

- 1 ⅓ cups olive oil
- ½ lb. salmon fillets
- 2 cups coconut milk, freshly squeezed
- 2 tbsp. curry powder
- 1 ¼ cups cilantro chopped
- Pepper and salt to taste

**Directions:**

1. In your instant pot, add in all ingredients. Apply a seasoning of pepper and salt. Give a good stir.
2. Set the lid in place and the vent to point to "Sealing."
3. Set the IP to "Manual" and cook for 10 minutes.
4. Do quick pressure release.

**Nutrition values per serving:**
Calories: 1783Kcal | Protein: 14.9g | Fat: 195.2g | Carbs: 17g

## 66. Seared Salmon with Braised Broccoli

**Preparation time:** 1 hour
**Cooking time:** 30 minutes
**Servings:** 4
**Ingredients:**

- ½ cups water
- 2 tbsp. pine nuts
- 3 tbsp. raisins
- 1 small onion, diced
- 1 ½ tbsp. extra-virgin olive oil, divided
- 2 heads broccoli, trimmed
- 1 tsp. salt, divided
- 1 tsp. dried or one tbsp. fresh rosemary; chopped and divided
- 1 ¼ lb. wild Alaskan salmon fillet, cut into four pieces

**Directions:**

1. Use a ½ tsp. salt and half of the rosemary to season the salmon for about 20–60 minutes. Also, cut into florets the broccoli with 2-inch-long stalks.
2. Using a vegetable peeler, remove the stalk's tough covering and cut the florets into half, lengthwise.
3. In a large and wide saucepan, heat 1 tbsp. oil over medium heat Add in onion and cook the mixture for about 3–4 minutes, until translucent.

4. Then add in the remaining rosemary, pine nuts, raisins, and toss to cover with oil. Continue to cook for 3–5 minutes to have the pine nuts turn fragrant and start to brown.
5. Add in broccoli and season with a ½ tsp. salt, tossing to combine. To this mixture, add in water, bring to boil, and then reduce the heat to maintain a simmer.
6. Cook for about 8–10 minutes, and stir regularly. Cook until most of the water has evaporated.
7. Into a large non-stick skillet, heat ½ tbsp. oil over medium heat. Add in the salmon, the skinned side facing up, and cook for 3–5 minutes to have it turn golden brown. Turn it over, remove the salmon from the heat, and slowly cook through for additional 3–5 minutes.
8. When done, sub-divide the broccoli into 4 plates and top with the salmon, pine nuts, spoon raisins, and other remaining liquid from the pan.

**Nutrition values per serving:**
Calories: 304Kcal | Protein: 29.8g | Fat: 17.1g | Carbs: 10.6g

## 67. Satisfying Turkey Lettuce Wraps

**Preparation time:** 15 minutes
**Cooking time:** 20 minutes
**Servings:** 4
**Ingredients:**

- ½ lb. ground turkey
- ½ small onion, finely chopped
- 1 garlic clove, minced
- 2 tbsp. extra virgin olive oil
- 1 head lettuce
- 1 tsp. cumin
- ½ tbsp. fresh ginger, sliced
- 2 tbsp. apple cider vinegar
- 2 tbsp. freshly chopped cilantro
- 1 tsp. freshly ground black pepper
- 1 tsp. sea salt

**Directions:**

1. Sauté garlic and onion in extra virgin olive oil until fragrant and translucent.
2. Add turkey and cook well.
3. Stir in the remaining ingredients and continue cooking for 5 minutes more.
4. To serve, ladle a spoonful of turkey mixture onto a lettuce leaf and wrap. Enjoy!

**Nutrition values per serving:**
Calories: 194Kcal | Protein: 16.3g | Fat: 13.6g | Carbs: 4.6g

## 68. White Bean & Veggie Salad

**Preparation time:** 10 minutes
**Cooking time:** 10 minutes
**Servings:** 1
**Ingredients:**

- 2 cups mixed salad greens
- ¾ cup veggies
- 1/3 cup canned white beans
- ½ avocado
- 1 tbsp. red wine vinegar
- 2 tsp. olive oil
- ¼ tsp. kosher salt
- Ground fresh pepper

**Directions:**

1. In a bowl, mix greens, beans, veggies, & avocado in a bowl. Drizzle it with vinegar, oil and season with salt and pepper. Toss it to combine & transfer it to a large plate.

**Nutrition values per serving:**
Calories: 360kcal | Proteins: 10.1g | Fats: 24.6g | Carbs: 29.7g

## 69. Greek Meatball Mezze Bowls

**Preparation time:** 35 minutes
**Cooking time:** 35 minutes
**Servings:** 4
**Ingredients:**

- 1 cup frozen chopped spinach
- 1 pound 93% lean ground turkey
- crumbled feta cheese ½ cup
- ½ tsp. garlic powder
- ½ tsp. dried oregano
- 3/8 tsp. salt
- 3/8 tsp. pepper, ground
- 2 cups quinoa, cooked
- 2 tbsp. lemon juice
- 1 tbsp. olive oil
- ½ cup parsley, chopped
- 3 tbsp. mint, chopped
- 2 cups sliced cucumber
- 1 pint cherry tomatoes
- ¼ cup tzatziki

**Directions:**

1. Squeeze out extra moisture from the spinach. Mix spinach with feta, garlic, turkey, oregano, salt, pepper, and mix them well. Make the

mixture in 12 meatballs. Heat a large skillet over medium heat.

2. Coat with cooking spray and add meatballs to the pan. Cook till browned from all sides & pink from the center for 10 minutes. Mix lemon juice, mint, parsley, oil, salt, pepper, and quinoa and top every meatball, cherry tomatoes and cucumbers in a single serving.
3. Packed up and refrigerate it for 4 days.
4. Divide tzatziki before serving and transfer meatballs in a safe oven to heat till steaming. Return to the original one and serve with tzatziki.

**Nutrition values per serving:**

Calories: 392kcal | Proteins: 32.4g | Fats: 17.2g | Carbs: 29.3g

## 70. Mediterranean Chickpea Quinoa Bowl

**Preparation time:** 20 minutes
**Cooking time:** 20 minutes
**Servings:** 4
**Ingredients:**

- 1 jar roasted red peppers
- ¼ cup silvered almonds
- 4 tbsp. olive oil
- 1 small garlic clove
- 1 tsp. paprika
- ½ tsp. ground cumin
- ¼ tsp. crushed red pepper
- 2 cups cooked quinoa
- ¼ cup kalamata olives
- ¼ cup chopped red onion
- 1 can chickpeas
- 1 cup diced cucumber
- ¼ cup crumbled feta cheese
- 2 tbsp. fresh parsley

**Directions:**

1. Put almonds, garlic, paprika, red pepper, cumin, oil, and peppers in a blender till smooth.
2. Mix red onion, oil, and quinoa in a bowl.
3. Divide the quinoa mixture into four bowls with equal chickpeas, red pepper sauce, and cucumber. Spray with feta and parsley.

**Nutrition values per serving:**

Calories: 479kcal | Proteins: 12.7g | Fats: 24.8g | Carbs: 49.5g

## 71. Tomato, Cucumber & White-Bean Salad with Basil Vinaigrette

**Preparation time:** 25 minutes
**Cooking time:** 25 minutes
**Servings:** 4
**Ingredients:**

- ½ cup fresh basil leaves
- ¼ cup olive oil
- 3 tbsp. red-wine vinegar
- 1 tbsp. finely chopped shallot
- 2 tsp. Dijon mustard
- 1 tsp. honey
- ¼ tsp. salt
- ¼ tsp. ground pepper
- 10 cups mixed salad greens
- 1 can cannellini beans
- 1 cup grape tomatoes
- 1/2 cucumber

**Directions:**

1. Put oil, basil, mustard, shallot, salt, honey, and pepper in a blender.
2. Process till become smooth and transfer to a bowl. Add greens, tomatoes, beans, and cucumber. Toss to coat.

**Nutrition values per serving:**

Calories: 246kcal | Proteins: 7.5g | Fats: 15.3g | Carbs: 21.5g

## 72. Tuna and Spinach Salad

**Preparation time:** 10 minutes
**Cooking time:** 10 minutes
**Servings:** 1
**Ingredients:**

- 1 ½ tbsp. tahini
- 1 ½ tbsp. lemon juice
- 1 ½ tbsp. water
- 1 can light tuna in water
- 4 kalamata olives
- 2 tbsp. feta cheese
- 2 tbsp. parsley
- 2 cups baby spinach
- 1 medium orange

**Directions:**

1. Mix tahini, water, and lemon juice in a bowl.

2. Add parsley, feta, tuna, olives, and mix well. Serve the tuna salad over 2 cups with oranges.

**Nutrition values per serving:**
Calories: 376kcal | Proteins: 25.7g | Fats: 21g | Carbs: 26.2g

## 73. Mozzarella, Basil, and Zucchini Frittata

**Preparation time:** 20 minutes
**Cooking time:** 20 minutes
**Servings:** 4
**Ingredients:**

- 2 tbsp. olive oil
- 1 ½ cups red onion
- 1 ½ cups zucchini
- 7 large eggs
- ½ tsp. salt
- ¼ tsp. ground pepper
- 2/3 cup pearl size mozzarella balls
- 3 tbsp. chopped sun-dried tomatoes
- ¼ cup fresh basil

**Directions:**

1. Put the rack on the upper third of the oven and heat the broiler.
2. Heat oil in a skillet on medium heat. Add onion, zucchini to it and cook for 3 to 5 minutes.
3. Mix eggs, pepper, salt in a bowl and pour the eggs on the veggies in the pan. Cook from the middle till set for 2 minutes.
4. Arrange mozzarella and tomatoes on top and place the skillet under the broiler till the eggs are browned for 2 minutes. Top it with basil.
5. Run a spatula around the edge to release the frittata from the pan and cut them into 4 slices.

**Nutrition values per serving:**
Calories: 292kcal | Proteins: 17.6g | Fats: 20.7g | Carbs: 7.8g

## 74. Spinach & Egg Scramble with Raspberries

**Preparation time:** 10 minutes
**Cooking time:** 10 minutes
**Servings:** 1
**Ingredients:**

- 1 tsp. canola oil
- 1 ½ cup baby spinach
- 2 large eggs
- Salt a pinch
- Ground pepper pinch
- 1 slice whole-grain bread
- ½ cup fresh raspberries

**Directions:**

1. Heat oil in a small skillet on medium heat. Add spinach and cook till wilted for 2 minutes.
2. Transfer the spinach to a plate. Add eggs after placing on medium heat. Cook till just set out and mix in salt, pepper, and spinach. Serve with raspberries.

**Nutrition values per serving:**
Calories: 296kcal | Proteins: 17.8g | Fats: 15.7g | Carbs: 20.9g

## 75. Chicken with Orzo Salad

**Preparation time:** 40 minutes
**Cooking time:** 40 minutes
**Servings:** 4
**Ingredients:**

- 2 boneless chicken breasts, skinless
- 3 tbsp. olive oil
- 1 tsp. lemon zest
- ½ tsp. salt
- ½ tsp. ground pepper
- ¾ cup whole-wheat orzo
- 2 cups baby spinach
- 1 cup chopped cucumber
- 1 cup chopped tomato
- ¼ cup chopped red onion
- ¼ cup crumbled feta cheese
- 2 tbsp. chopped kalamata olives
- 2 tbsp. lemon juice
- 1 garlic clove
- 2 tsp. chopped fresh oregano

**Directions:**

1. Heat the oven to 425 degrees F.
2. Brush chicken with oil and spray lemon zest, salt, and pepper. Put in a baking dish and bake till the thermometer inserted in the thickest part shows 165 degrees F for 30 minutes.
3. Add in quarter warm water orzo and cook for 8 minutes. Add spinach for 1 minute. Drain and rinse it with cold water. Drain well and transfer it to a bowl. Add onion, tomato, olives, feta, and cucumber and mix it well.

4. Whisk the remaining oregano, oil, garlic, lemon juice, pepper, and salt in a bowl. Stir it into the orzo mixture. Drizzle it with dressing on the chicken and serve with the salad.

**Nutrition values per serving:**

Calories: 402kcal | Proteins: 32g | Fats: 7.5g | Carbs: 28.3g

## 76. Mason Jar Power Salad with Chickpeas & Tuna

**Preparation time:** 5 minutes
**Cooking time:** 5 minutes
**Servings:** 1
**Ingredients:**

- 3 cups chopped kale
- 2 tbsp. honey mustard vinaigrette
- 1 2.5-ounce tuna in water
- ½ cup rinsed canned chickpeas
- 1 shredded carrot

**Directions:**

1. Toss dressing and kale in a bowl. Transfer in a mason jar. Top it with tuna, chickpeas, and carrot. Refrigerate it for 2 days.
2. Empty the jar contents in a bowl after serving and combine it well with salad ingredients and the dressed kale.

**Nutrition values per serving:**

Calories: 430kcal | Proteins: 26.4g | Fats: 22.7g | Carbs: 30.1g

## 77. Creamy Pesto Chicken Salad with Greens

**Preparation time:** 30 minutes
**Cooking time:** 30 minutes
**Servings:** 4
**Ingredients:**

- 1 pound chicken breasts
- ¼ cup pesto
- ¼ cup low-fat mayonnaise
- 3 tbsp. chopped red onion
- 3 tbsp. olive oil
- 2 tbsp. red wine vinegar
- ¼ tsp. salt
- ¼ tsp. ground pepper
- 1 5-ounce package mixed salad greens
- 1 pint cherry tomatoes

**Directions:**

1. Put chicken in a saucepan and add water to bring it to a simmer point. Cover it and lower down the heat till pink from the middle for 15 minutes. Transfer it to clean the cutting board after cooling down.
2. Mix mayonnaise, onion, and pesto in a bowl. Add the chicken & toss to coat. Mix vinegar, pepper, salt, oil in a bowl.
3. Add tomatoes and greens and toss to coat. Divide the green salad among 4 plates and top it with chicken salad.

**Nutrition values per serving:**

Calories: 324kcal | Proteins: 27.1g | Fats: 19.7g | Carbs: 9.2g

## 78. Chicken Quinoa Bowl

**Preparation time:** 30 minutes
**Cooking time:** 30 minutes
**Servings:** 4
**Ingredients:**

- 1 pound chicken breasts
- ¼ tsp. salt
- ¼ tsp. ground pepper
- 1 7-ounce roasted red peppers
- ¼ cup silvered almonds
- 4 tbsp. olive oil
- 1 small garlic clove
- 1 tsp. paprika
- ½ tsp. ground cumin
- ¼ tsp. crushed red pepper, optional
- 2 cups cooked quinoa
- ¼ cups kalamata olives
- ¼ cup chopped red onion
- 1 cup diced cucumber
- ¼ cup feta crumbled cheese
- 2 tbsp. chopped fresh parsley

**Directions:**

1. Put in a rack of oven third part after heating broiler at high heat. Line a baking sheet with foil.
2. Spray chicken with pepper and salt. Place on the prepared baking sheet. Broil till the thermometer inserted in the thickest part reads 165 degrees F for 16 minutes. Transfer the chicken to a clean cutting board and slice it.
3. Place peppers, oil, garlic, paprika, almonds, cumin, and red pepper in a blender. Puree till smooth.

4. Mix olives, red onion, and quinoa in an oiled bowl. Divide the quinoa mixture into four bowls and top it with equal amounts of cucumber for serving. Spray with feta and parsley.

**Nutrition values per serving:**

Calories: 519kcal | Proteins: 34.1g | Fats: 26.9g | Carbs: 31.2g

## 79. Greek Chicken & Cucumber Pita with Yogurt Sauce

**Preparation time:** 45 minutes
**Cooking time:** 1 hour 45 minutes
**Servings:** 4
**Ingredients:**

- 1 tsp. lemon zest
- 2 tbsp. fresh lemon juice
- 5 tsp. olive oil
- 1 tbsp. fresh oregano chopped
- 1 ¾ tsp. minced garlic
- ¼ tsp. crushed red pepper
- 1 pound chicken tenders
- 1 English cucumber
- ½ tsp. salt
- ¾ cup Greek yogurt
- 2 tsp. chopped fresh mint
- 2 tsp. chopped fresh dill
- 1 tsp. ground pepper
- 2 whole-wheat pita bread
- 4 lettuce leaves
- ½ cup sliced red onion
- 1 cup chopped plum tomatoes

**Directions:**

1. Mix lemon zest, juice, oregano, garlic, red pepper, and oil in a bowl. Add chicken and toss to coat.
2. Marinate in the refrigerator for almost 4 hours. Toss cucumber, salt, sieve, and let it drain for 15 minutes. Squeeze out the liquid and transfer it to a medium bowl. Mix in yogurt, dill, pepper, oil, salt, garlic, mint, and refrigerate till serving.
3. Heat the grill to medium level. Oil the grill rack and grill the chicken till a thermometer is inserted in the center at 165 degrees F for 4 minutes per side.
4. Sprinkle some sauce on every side for serving.

**Nutrition values per serving:**

Calories: 353kcal | Proteins: 37.5g | Fats: 8.6g | Carbs: 33.3g

## 80. Harissa Chickpea Stew with Eggplant and Millet

**Preparation time:** 35 minutes
**Cooking time:** 10 minutes
**Servings:** 2
**Ingredients:**

- 1 cup millet
- Kosher salt
- 2 tbsp. ghee
- 1 large Japanese eggplant
- Black pepper freshly ground
- 1 diced onion
- 3 garlic cloves, minced
- 1 14-ounce can tomato puree
- 1 14-ounce can chickpeas drained
- 2 tbsp. harissa pastes
- 1 bunch cilantro for garnish

**Directions:**

1. Fill a saucepan with water and add the millet with a salt pinch. Bring to a boil and cover it. Reduce the heat and cook for 25 minutes. After the millet cooking is done, remove the lid and fluff it with a fork and allow it to cool.
2. Heat oil in a skillet on medium heat. Add the salt, pepper, eggplant, and cook till golden and tender. Add some more oil and cook for 10 minutes. Transfer the eggplant to a bowl and set it aside.
3. Add the leftover oil to the same skillet and add onion to it. Cook till soft and golden brown for 10 minutes.
4. Add the garlic and cook for 2 minutes. Season it with pepper and salt. Add the tomatoes, harissa, and chickpeas and return to the skillet after reducing the heat to low. Allow it to simmer for 15 minutes. Divide the millet between 2 bowls and top it with stew.

**Nutrition values per serving:**

Calories: 600kcal | Proteins: 20g | Fats: 15g | Carbs: 100g

## 81. Grilled Lemon-Herb Chicken & Avocado Salad

**Preparation time:** 35 minutes
**Cooking time:** 1 hour
**Servings:** 4

**Ingredients:**

- Lemon-Herb Chicken
- 1½ pounds chicken breasts, boneless and skinless
- 3 tbsp. olive oil
- Zest & juice of 2 lemons
- 1 tbsp. chopped fresh oregano
- 1 tbsp. chopped fresh dill
- 3 tbsp. chopped fresh parsley
- Kosher salt & black pepper

Salad

- 1 cup barley
- 2½ cups chicken broth
- zest & juice of 1 lemon
- 1 tbsp. whole-grain mustard
- 1 tsp. dried oregano
- ⅓ cup olive oil
- Kosher salt & black pepper
- 2 chopped heads of red-leaf lettuce
- 1 halved and thinly sliced red onion
- 1 pint sliced cherry tomatoes
- 2 sliced avocados

**Directions:**

1. Put chicken in a plastic bag and mix olive oil, lemon juice, and zest, dill, oregano, parsley in it and marinade into that bag. Refrigerate for 29 – 30 minutes. Bring the chicken and barley in a saucepan and simmer on medium heat. Cover the pot and cook till the barley is tender for 45 minutes. Drain and reserve. Mix the lemon juice, zest, mustard, oregano in a bowl. Mix well and season it with salt & pepper.
2. Prepare the grill at high heat and remove the chicken from the marinade. Season it with salt and pepper. Grill the chicken and be well-charged from both sides and cooked completely. Flipping them as needed and remove them from the grill, and reserve. Toss the onion, lettuce and tomatoes in a bowl. Add the dressing and toss to coat.
3. Slice the chicken and serve them at the top of the salad.

**Nutrition values per serving:**

Calories: 309kcal | Proteins: 39g | Fats: 15g | Carbs: 4g

## 82. Minute Heirloom Tomato and Cucumber Toast

**Preparation time:** 5 minutes
**Cooking time:** 0 minutes
**Servings:** 1
**Ingredients:**

- 1 small diced heirloom tomato
- 1 diced Persian cucumber
- 1 tsp. olive oil
- A pinch dried oregano
- Kosher salt & black pepper
- 2 tsp. whipped cream cheese
- 2 pieces of trader joe's crispbread, whole grain
- 1 tsp. balsamic glaze

**Directions:**

1. Mix cucumber, olive oil, tomato, and oregano, with salt & pepper in a bowl.
2. Smear the cream cheese on the bread and top it with the cucumber-tomato mixture and the balsamic glaze.

**Nutrition values per serving:**

Calories: 177kcal | Proteins: 3g | Fats: 8g | Carbs: 24g

## 83. Greek Chicken and Rice Skillet

**Preparation time:** 15 minutes
**Cooking time:** 25 minutes
**Servings:** 4-6
**Ingredients:**

- 6 chicken thighs
- Kosher salt & black pepper
- 1 tsp. dried oregano
- 1 tsp. garlic powder
- 3 lemons
- 2 tbsp. olive oil
- ½ red onion, minced
- 2 garlic cloves, minced
- 1 cup long-grain rice
- 2½ cups chicken broth
- 1 tbsp. chopped fresh oregano
- 1 cup green olives
- ½ cup crumbled feta cheese
- ⅓ cup chopped fresh parsley

**Directions:**

1. Heat the oven to 375 degrees F. season chicken thighs with pepper and salt. Mix the dried oregano, lemon zest, and garlic powder in a bowl.
2. Heat the olive oil in a skillet on medium heat. Add the chickpea, and sear it until the chicken is browned for 9 minutes. Remove from a plate and reserve.
3. Add garlic and onions in the skillet and sauté till translucent for 5 minutes and mix in the rice for 1 min with salt.
4. Add the chicken broth and bring it to the mixture and simmer it. Mix the fresh oregano and lemon juice, zest, and slice down the remaining 2 lemons. Set them aside. Nestle chicken into the rice mixture. Transfer the skillet to the oven and cook till the rice has absorbed all the liquid. Chicken becomes completely cooked for 25 minutes. Turn on the broiler and arrange the lemon slices on the chicken. Broil it to the skillet until the lemons are charred and chicken skin becomes crisp for 3 minutes.
5. Add feta and olives to the skillet and garnish it with fresh parsley. Serve immediately.

**Nutrition values per serving:**
Calories: 903kcal | Proteins: 48g | Fats: 55g | Carbs: 54g

## 84. Mini Chicken Shawarma

**Preparation time:** 1 hour 10 minutes
**Cooking time:** 30 minutes
**Servings:** 8
**Ingredients:**
Chicken
- 1 pound chicken tenders
- ¼ cup olive oil
- Zest & juice of 1 lemon
- 2 tsp. garlic powder
- 1 tsp. ground cumin
- ¾ tsp. ground coriander
- ½ tsp. smoked paprika
- 1 tsp. ground black pepper

Sauce
- 1¼ cups Greek yogurt
- 1 tbsp. lemon juice
- 1 garlic clove, grated
- ¼ cup chopped fresh parsley
- 2 tbsp. chopped fresh dill
- Kosher salt & black pepper
- ½ red onion, thinly sliced
- 4 leaves romaine lettuce, shredded
- ½ English cucumber, thinly sliced
- 2 tomatoes, chopped - 16 mini pita bread

**Directions:**

1. Put chicken in a plastic bag. Mix olive oil, garlic powder, lemon juice, zest, paprika, cumin, coriander, and pepper in a bowl. Pour the marinade in that bag and toss to coat. Let the chicken marinate for 30 minutes to 1 hr. Stir the lemon juice, zest, garlic, and yogurt in a bowl during the marinated chicken time. Stir in the parsley and dill with salt and pepper. Cover it and refrigerate it.
2. Heat a skillet on medium heat and remove the chicken from the marinade. Mix the marinade and remove the chicken and cook till browned from both sides for 4 minutes. Chop them into strips. Divide the chicken, onion, cucumber, lettuce, tomato to assemble.

**Nutrition values per serving:**
Calories: 216kcal | Proteins: 9g | Fats: 16g | Carbs: 10g

## 85. 15-Minute Couscous with Tuna & Pepperoncini

**Preparation time:** 3 minutes
**Cooking time:** 12 minutes
**Servings:** 4
**Ingredients:**
Couscous
- 1 cup chicken broth
- 1¼ cups couscous
- ¾ tsp. kosher salt

Accompaniments
- two 5-ounce cans of oil-packed tuna
- 1 pint cherry tomatoes, halved
- ½ cup sliced pepperoncini
- ⅓ cup chopped fresh parsley
- ¼ cup capers
- Olive oil, for serving
- Kosher salt & black pepper
- 1 lemon, quartered

**Directions:**

1. Bring the broth to a boiling point on medium heat. Remove it from the heat and stir and cover the pot. Let it down for 10 minutes.
2. Toss the tuna, tomatoes, capers, parsley, and pepperoncini in a bowl.
3. Fluff the couscous by using a fork and season it with salt and pepper. Drizzle with olive oil and

top with the couscous along with tuna mixture. Serve it with lemon wedges.

**Nutrition values per serving:**

Calories: 226kcal | Proteins: 8g | Fats: 1g | Carbs: 44g

## 86. Pesto Quinoa Bowls with Roasted Veggies and Labneh

**Preparation time:** 10 minutes
**Cooking time:** 40 minutes
**Servings:** 4
**Ingredients:**

- 1 large Japanese eggplant, cubed
- 1 medium zucchini, cubed
- 1 pint cherry tomatoes
- A handful of Romano beans
- olive oil
- kosher salt & black pepper
- 1 cup quinoa, rinsed
- ½ cup pesto
- 1 cup labneh or Greek yogurt
- 1 garlic clove, minced
- ½ lemon juice
- Cilantro or parsley handful

**Directions:**

1. Heat the oven to 400 degrees F and line a baking sheet with parchment paper. Arrange the zucchini, tomatoes, eggplant, and beans on it. Drizzle the olive oil on the veggies and season it with salt & pepper. Roast till all the veggies become softened and caramelized, for 30 to 40 minutes.
2. Add quinoa in a saucepan along with water and a pinch of salt. Bring to a boil and simmer and cook it for 15 minutes. After cooking the quinoa, remove the lid and fluff by using a fork. Allow it to cool down. Mix lemon juice, zest, herbs, and labneh in a bowl.
3. Assemble every bowl after adding quinoa and arranging the veggies in rows just like a rainbow. Add a dollop of the labneh on the side.

**Nutrition values per serving:**

Calories: 862kcal | Proteins: 32g | Fats: 42g | Carbs: 96g

## 87. Greek Yogurt Chicken Salad with Stuffed Peppers

**Preparation time:** 30 minutes
**Cooking time:** 0 minutes
**Servings:** 6
**Ingredients:**

- ⅔ cup Greek yogurt
- 2 tbsp. Dijon mustard
- 2 tbsp. seasoned rice vinegar
- Kosher salt & black pepper
- ⅓ cup chopped fresh parsley
- Meat from 1 rotisserie chicken, cubed
- 4 stalks celery, sliced
- 1 bunch scallions, sliced and divided
- 1 pint cherry tomatoes
- ½ cucumber, diced
- 3 bell peppers

**Directions:**

1. Mix the Greek yogurt, rice vinegar, salt, pepper, and mustard in a bowl. Stir in the parsley. Mix it well.
2. Add the celery, scallions, tomatoes, cucumbers, and chicken and mix it well.
3. Divide the chicken salad among bell pepper boats and garnish it with the leftover scallions, cucumbers, and tomatoes.

**Nutrition values per serving:**

Calories: 400kcal | Proteins: 60g | Fats: 10g | Carbs: 17g

## 88. Chicken Skewers with Tzatziki Sauce

**Preparation time:** 30 minutes
**Cooking time:** 1 hour
**Servings:** 6
**Ingredients:**

Tzatziki sauce

- 1 cup Greek yogurt
- ½ European cucumber, diced
- 1 tbsp. olive oil
- 2 tbsp. lemon juice
- A pinch of garlic powder
- Salt & black pepper
- ¼ cup fresh chopped dill

Skewers

- ¼ cup Greek yogurt
- Zest & juice of 1 lemon
- 1 tsp. dried oregano
- 1 tsp. garlic powder
- A pinch of cayenne pepper
- 1 ½ pounds chicken breast boneless skinless
- Olive oil, as needed

- Salt & black pepper
- ¼ cup chopped fresh parsley

**Directions:**
1. Mix yogurt with olive oil, garlic powder, lemon juice, and cucumber in a bowl. Mix it well and season it with salt and pepper. Mix the yogurt with oregano, garlic powder, cayenne, lemon juice, and zest in a bowl.
2. Rub chicken with the above mixture to coat it well in another bowl. Put one piece of chicken on every skewer and brush the skewers from both sides with olive oil. Season with salt and pepper on a preheated grill for 5 minutes.
3. Serve immediately and garnish it with parsley and tzatziki sauce.

**Nutrition values per serving:**
Calories: 68kcal | Proteins: 4g | Fats: 5g | Carbs: 3g

## 89. "Zoodles Salad"

**Preparation time:** 20 minutes
**Cooking time:** 0 minutes
**Servings:** 4
**Ingredients:**
- 1 lemon
- ½ tsp. Dijon mustard
- ½ tsp. garlic powder
- ⅓ cup olive oil
- Salt & black pepper
- 3 medium zucchini, cut into noodles
- 1 bunch radishes, thinly sliced
- 1 tbsp. chopped fresh thyme

**Directions:**
1. Mix mustard, lemon juice, zest, garlic powder in a bowl.
2. Add the olive oil slowly and mix it well. Season it with salt and pepper.
3. Toss the zucchini noodles and the radishes in another bowl and add the dressing to coat it well.
4. Serve immediately and garnish with fresh thyme.

**Nutrition values per serving:**
Calories: 198kcal | Proteins: 2g | Fats: 19g | Carbs: 8g

## 90. Mediterranean Quinoa Bowls

**Preparation time:** 15 minutes
**Cooking time:** 5 minutes
**Servings:** 8
**Ingredients:**
- red pepper roasted sauce
- 16 oz. red pepper, roasted
- 1 garlic clove
- ½ tsp. salt
- 1 lemon juice
- ½ cup olive oil
- ½ cup almonds

For bowls (Create your own bowls depending on your tastes)
- spinach
- cooked quinoa
- kalamata olives
- feta cheese
- red onion
- pepperoncini
- basil or parsley
- hummus
- lemon juice
- pepper & salt
- olive oil

**Directions:**
1. Mix all ingredients in a blender till smooth. Cook the quinoa according to the instructions given on the package. When quinoa is made, the Mediterranean bowls are made. Serve with greens and sauces.

**Nutrition values per serving:**
Calories: 381kcal | Proteins: 10.9g | Fats: 25.6g | Carbs: 30.9g

## 91. Greek Lemon Chicken Soup

**Preparation time:** 10 minutes
**Cooking time:** 20 minutes
**Servings:** 6
**Ingredients:**
- 1 tbsp. olive oil
- 1 pound chicken thighs
- Salt & pepper
- 4 garlic cloves
- 1 onion
- 3 carrots
- 2 celery stalks
- ½ tsp. dried thyme
- 8 cups chicken stock
- 2 bay leaves

- 1 can cannellini beans
- 4 cups baby spinach
- 2 tbsp. lemon juice
- 2 tbsp. fresh parsley
- 2 tbsp. fresh dill

**Directions:**
1. Heat olive oil in an oven at medium heat.
2. Season chicken with pepper and salt. Add chicken to the Dutch oven and cook till golden for 3 minutes.
3. Add garlic, celery, carrots, and onion and cook till tender for 3 minutes. Mix it well for 1 min.
4. Mix in chicken stock & bay leaves. Bring to a boil and lower the heat. Stir frequently for 10 to 15 minutes.
5. Mix well in spinach till wilted for 2 minutes. Mix it well in lemon juice, dill, and parsley. Season it with salt and pepper. Serve immediately.

**Nutrition values per serving:**

Calories: 241kcal | Proteins: 19g | Fats: 9g | Carbs: 18g

## 92. Stuffed Eggplant

**Preparation time:** 10 minutes
**Cooking time:** 40 minutes
**Servings:** 4
**Ingredients:**
- 2 medium eggplants
- 2 tbsp. olive oil
- 1 red onion
- 2 garlic cloves
- 1 pint cremini mushrooms
- 2 cups torn kale
- 2 cups cooked quinoa
- 1 tbsp. fresh thyme
- Juice and zest of 1 lemon
- Salt & pepper
- ½ cup Greek yogurt
- Fresh parsley 3 tbsp.

**Directions:**
1. Heat the oven to 400 degrees F. Line a baking sheet along with parchment paper.
2. Scoop out the flesh of eggplant by using a spoon and rub inside with olive oil. Transfer it to the prepared baking sheet.
3. Add olive oil to a skillet and heat it to a medium level. Add onion and sauté till soft for 4 minutes. Add garlic now and cook for 1 more min.
4. Add mushrooms and cook till 5 minutes. Mix kale & quinoa and cook for 3 minutes. Season it with thyme, salt, pepper, and zest.
5. Roast the eggplant after spooning the filling of prepared eggplants till soft for 20 minutes. Let them cool for 5 minutes. Serve immediately.

**Nutrition values per serving:**

Calories: 339kcal | Proteins: 12g | Fats: 15g | Carbs: 46g

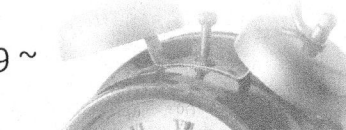

# CHAPTER 13

# Dinner

## 93. Garlic and Herb Grilled Chicken Breast

**Preparation time:** 7 minutes
**Cooking time:** 20 minutes
**Servings:** 4
**Ingredients:**

- 1 ¼ lb. chicken breasts, skinless and boneless
- 2 tsp. olive oil
- 1 tbsp. garlic & herb seasoning blend
- Salt
- Pepper

**Directions:**

1. Pat dry the chicken breasts, coat it with olive oil, and season it with salt and pepper on both sides.
2. Season the chicken with garlic and herb seasoning or any other seasoning of your choice.
3. Turn the grill on and oil the grate.
4. Place the chicken on the hot grate and let it grill till the sides turn white.
5. Flip them over and let them cook again.
6. When the internal temperature is about 160°F, it is most likely cooked.
7. Set aside for 15 minutes. Chop into pieces.

**Nutrition values per serving:**
Calories: 289Kcal | Protein: 41g | Fat: 12.8g | Carbs: 0g

## 94. Cajun Shrimp

**Preparation time:** 10 minutes
**Cooking time:** 5 minutes
**Servings:** 2
**Ingredients:**

- 16 tiger shrimp
- 2 tbsp. corn starch
- 1 tsp. cayenne pepper
- 1 tsp. old bay seasoning
- 1 tsp. olive oil
- Salt
- Pepper

**Directions:**

1. Rinse the shrimp. Pat dry.
2. In a bowl, combine corn starch, cayenne pepper, old bay seasoning, salt, and pepper. Stir it.
3. In a bowl, add the shrimp. Drizzle olive oil over shrimp to lightly coat.
4. Dip the shrimp in seasoning, shake off any excess.
5. Preheat fryer to 375°F. Lightly spray cook basket with non-stick keto cooking spray.
6. Transfer to the fryer. Cook 5 minutes; shake after 2 minutes, until cooked thoroughly.
7. Serve on a platter.

**Nutrition values per serving:**
Calories: 956Kcal | Protein: 189.8g | Fat: 12.3g | Carbs: 9.5g

## 95. Sesame-Crusted Mahi-Mahi

**Preparation time:** 5 minutes
**Cooking time:** 13 minutes
**Servings:** 4
**Ingredients:**

- 2 tbsp. Dijon mustard
- 1 tbsp. sour cream, low-fat
- ½ cup sesame seeds
- 2 tbsp. olive oil
- 1 lemon, wedged
- 4 (4 oz. each) mahi-mahi or sole filets

**Directions:**

1. Rinse filets and pat dry. In a bowl, mix sour cream and mustard. Spread this mixture on all sides of the fish Roll in sesame seeds to coat.
2. Heat olive oil in a large skillet over medium heat. Pan-fry fish, turning once, for 5–8 minutes or until fish flakes when tested with fork and sesame seeds are toasted. Serve immediately with lemon wedges.

**Nutrition values per serving:**
Calories: 305Kcal | Protein: 30.8g | Fat: 18g | Carbs: 6.7g

## 96. Country Chicken

**Preparation time:** 10 minutes
**Cooking time:** 15 minutes
**Servings:** 2
**Ingredients:**

- ¾ lb. chicken tenders, fresh, boneless skinless
- ½ cup almond meal
- ½ cup almond flour
- 1 tsp. rosemary, dried
- Salt
- Pepper
- 2 eggs, beaten

**Directions:**

1. Rinse the chicken tenders, pat dry.
2. In a medium bowl, pour in almond flour.
3. In a medium bowl, beat the eggs.
4. In a separate bowl, pour in an almond meal Season with rosemary, salt, and pepper.
5. Take the chicken pieces and toast in flour, then egg, then almond meal. Set on a tray.
6. Place the tray in the freezer for 5 minutes.
7. Preheat fryer to 350°F. Lightly spray cook basket with non-stick cooking spray.
8. Cook tenders for 10 minutes. After the timer runs out, set the temperature to 390°F, cook for 5 more minutes until golden brown.
9. Serve on a platter Side with preferred dipping sauce.

**Nutrition values per serving:**
Calories: 566Kcal | Protein: 61.3g | Fat: 32.4g | Carbs: 7.3g

## 97. Mahi-Mahi Tacos with Avocado and Fresh Cabbage

**Preparation time:** 5 minutes
**Cooking time:** 15 minutes
**Servings:** 4
**Ingredients:**

- 1 lb. mahi-mahi
- Salt
- Pepper
- 1 tsp. olive oil
- 1 avocado
- 4 corn tortillas
- 2 cups cabbage, shredded
- 2 quartered limes

**Directions:**

1. Season fish with salt and pepper.
2. Set a pan over medium-high heat. Add in oil and heat. Once the oil is hot, sauté fish for about 3–4 minutes on each side. Slice or flake fish into 1-oz. pieces.
3. Slice avocado in half. Remove seed and, using a spoon, remove the flesh from the skin. Slice the avocado halves into ½ thick slices.
4. In a small pan, warm corn tortillas; cook for about 1 minute on each side.
5. Place one-fourth of Mahi-mahi of each tortilla, top with avocado and cabbage. Serve with lime wedges.

**Nutrition values per serving:**
Calories: 298Kcal | Protein: 29.7g | Fat: 12.7g | Carbs: 17.1g

## 98. Butternut Squash Risotto

**Preparation time:** 10 minutes
**Cooking time:** 15 minutes
**Servings:** 4
**Ingredients:**

- 3 tbsp. butter
- 2 tbsp. minced sage
- ¼ tsp. black pepper, ground
- 1 tsp. minced rosemary
- 1 tsp. salt
- ½ cup dry sherry
- 4 cups riced cauliflower
- ½ cup butternut squash, cooked and mashed
- ½ cup parmesan cheese, grated
- ½ cup mascarpone cheese
- 1/8 tsp. grated nutmeg
- 1 tsp. minced garlic

**Directions:**

1. Melt your butter inside of a large frying pan turned to a medium level of heat.
2. Add your rosemary, your sage, and the garlic. Cook this for about 1 minute or until this mixture begins to become fragrant.
3. Add in the cauliflower rice, pepper and salt, and the mashed squash. Cook this for 3 minutes. You will know it is ready for the next step when cauliflower is starting to soften up for you.
4. Add in your sherry and cook this for an additional 6 minutes, or until the majority of the liquid is absorbed into the rice or when the cauliflower is much softer.
5. Stir in the mascarpone cheese, the parmesan cheese, as well as the nutmeg (grated).
6. Cook all of this on a medium heat level, being sure to stir it occasionally and do this until the cheese has melted and the risotto has gotten creamy. This will take around 4–5 minutes.

7. Taste the risotto and add more pepper and salt to season if you wish.
8. Remove your pan from the burner and garnish your risotto with more of the herbs as well as some grated parmesan.
9. Serve and enjoy!

**Nutrition values per serving:**

Calories: 188Kcal | Protein: 7g | Fat: 13.7g | Carbs: 9.6g

## 99. Cheesy Broccoli Soup

**Preparation time:** 5 minutes
**Cooking time:** 30 minutes
**Servings:** 2
**Ingredients:**

- 2 lb. broccoli, chopped
- Salt to taste
- 5 cups vegetable broth
- ¼ cup shredded cheddar cheese
- 1 tbsp. olive oil
- ¼ cup lemon juice
- 2 garlic cloves, mince
- 1 white onion, chopped
- Pepper to taste

**Directions:**

1. Heat the olive oil in a pan with medium heat. Fry the onion for 1 minute and then add the garlic. Fry until the garlic becomes golden in color.
2. Toss in the broccoli and stir for 3 minutes. Pour in the vegetable broth. Add salt, pepper and mix well. Cook for 20 minutes or until your broccoli is perfectly cooked through.
3. Take off the heat and let it cool down a bit. Add to a blender, and blend it until your soup is perfectly smooth.
4. Transfer the soup into the pot again and heat it over medium heat. Add lemon juice, cheddar cheese, and check if it needs a little more seasoning. Serve hot with more cheese on top.

**Nutrition values per serving:**

Calories: 401Kcal | Protein: 29.4g | Fat: 16.9g | Carbs: 39.4g

## 100. Beef Cabbage Stew

**Preparation time:** 30 minutes
**Cooking time:** 2 hours
**Servings:** 2
**Ingredients:**

- 2 lb. beef stew meat
- 1 cube beef bouillon
- 8-oz. tomato sauce
- ¼ cup chopped celery
- 2 bay leaves
- 8-oz. plum tomatoes, chopped
- 1 1/3 cups hot chicken broth
- Salt and pepper to taste
- 1 cabbage
- 1 tsp. Greek seasoning
- 4 onions, chopped

**Directions:**

1. Cut off the stem of the cabbage. Separate the leaves carefully. Wash well and rinse off. Set aside for now.
2. Fry the beef in a large pan over medium-low heat for about 8–10 minutes or until you get a brown color.
3. Into the pan, pour in 1/3 of the chicken broth.
4. Add the beef bouillon, and mix well.
5. Add the black pepper, salt and mix again.
6. Add the lid and cook on medium-low heat for about 1 hour.
7. Take off the heat and transfer the mix into a bowl.
8. Spread the cabbage leaves on a flat surface. Fill the middle using the beef mixture. Use a generous portion of filling; it will give your stew a better taste. Wrap the cabbage leaves tightly. Use a kitchen thread to tie it. Finish it with the remaining leaves and filling.
9. In a pot heat the oil over fry the onion for 1 minute.
10. Add the remaining chicken broth.
11. Add in the celery and tomato sauce and cook for another 10 minutes.
12. Add the Greek seasonings, and mix well. Bring to boil and then carefully add the wrapped cabbage. Cover and cook for another 10 minutes. Serve hot.

**Nutrition values per serving:**

Calories: 1023Kcal | Protein: 148.1g | Fat: 30.5g | Carbs: 31.9g

## 101. Fried Whole Tilapia

**Preparation time:** 10 minutes
**Cooking time:** 25 minutes
**Servings:** 2
**Ingredients:**

- 10-oz. tilapia
- 2 tbsp. olive oil
- 5 garlic cloves, mince
- 4 large onions, chopped
- 2 tbsp. red chili powder
- 1 tsp. turmeric powder

- 1 tsp. cumin powder
- 1 tsp. coriander powder
- Salt to taste
- Black pepper to taste
- 2 tbsp. soy sauce
- 2 tbsp. fish sauce

**Directions:**
1. Take the tilapia fish and clean it well without taking off the skin. You need to fry it whole, so you have to be careful about cleaning the gut inside.
2. Cut few slits on the skin, so the seasoning gets inside well.
3. Marinate the fish with fish sauce, soy sauce, red chili powder, cumin powder, turmeric powder, coriander powder, salt, and pepper.
4. Coat half of the onions in the same mixture too.
5. Let them marinate for 1 hour.
6. Heat the oil in a skillet. Fry the fish for 8 minutes on each side.
7. Transfer the fish to a serving plate.
8. Fry the marinated onions until they become crispy.
9. Add the remaining raw onions on top and serve hot.

**Nutrition values per serving:**
Calories: 414Kcal | Protein: 33.3g | Fat: 16.8g | Carbs: 37.7g

## 102. African Chicken Curry

**Preparation time:** 10 minutes
**Cooking time:** 30 minutes
**Servings:** 4
**Ingredients:**
- 1 lb. whole chicken
- ½ onion
- ½ cups coconut milk
- ½ bay leaf
- 1 ½ tsp. olive oil
- ½ cup peeled tomatoes
- 1 tsp. curry powder
- 1/8 tsp. salt
- ½ lemon, juiced
- 1 clove garlic

**Directions:**
1. Keep the skin of the chicken.
2. Cut your chicken into 8 pieces. It looks good when you keep the size not too small or not too big.
3. Discard the skin of the onion and garlic and mince the garlic and dice the onion.
4. Cut the tomato wedges.
5. Now in a pot, add the olive oil and heat over medium heat.
6. Add the garlic and fry until it becomes brown.
7. Add the diced onion and caramelize it.
8. Add the bay leaf and chicken pieces.
9. Fry the chicken pieces until they are golden.
10. Add the curry powder, coconut milk, and salt.
11. Cover and cook for 10 minutes on high heat.
12. Lower the heat to medium-low and add the lemon juice.
13. Add the tomato wedges and coconut milk. Cook for another 10 minutes.
14. Serve hot with rice or tortilla.

**Nutrition values per serving:**
Calories: 299Kcal | Protein: 34.1g | Fat: 15.7g | Carbs: 5.1g

## 103. Yummy Garlic Chicken Livers

**Preparation time:** 10 minutes
**Cooking time:** 30 minutes
**Servings:** 2
**Ingredients:**
- ½ lb. chicken liver
- 2 tsp. lime juice
- 6 garlic cloves, mince
- ½ tsp. salt
- 1 tbsp. ginger-garlic paste
- 1 cup diced onion
- 1 tbsp. red chili powder
- 1 tsp. cumin
- 1 tsp. coriander powder
- black pepper to taste
- 1 cardamom
- 2 tomatoes
- 1 cinnamon stick
- 1 bay leaf
- 4 tbsp. olive oil

**Directions:**
1. In a large pan, heat your oil over high heat.
2. Add the garlic and fry them golden brown.
3. Add onion and fry until they become caramelized.
4. Turn the heat to medium and add the bay leaf, cinnamon stick, cardamom, and toss for 30 seconds.
5. Add the ginger-garlic paste and 1 tbsp. water. Adding water prevents burning.
6. Add the coriander powder, black pepper, salt, cumin, and red chili powder.

7. Cover and cook for 3 minutes on low heat. Add the livers and cook on medium heat for 15 minutes.
8. Add the tomatoes and cook for another 5 minutes. Check the seasoning; add more salt if needed.
9. Serve hot with the tortilla.

**Nutrition values per serving:**
Calories: 554Kcal | Protein: 31.1g | Fat: 41g | Carbs: 18.8g

## 104. Healthy Chickpea Burger

**Preparation time:** 15 minutes
**Cooking time:** 10 minutes
**Servings:** 2
**Ingredients:**

- 1 cup chickpeas, boiled
- 1 tbsp. tomato puree
- 1 tsp. soy sauce
- A pinch paprika
- A pinch of white pepper
- 1 onion, diced
- Salt to taste
- 2 lettuce leaves
- ½ cups bell pepper, sliced
- 1 tsp. olive oil
- 1 avocado, sliced
- 2 burger buns to serve

**Directions:**
1. Mash the chickpeas and combine with bell pepper, salt, pepper, paprika, soy sauce, and tomato puree.
2. Use your hands to make patties.
3. Fry the patties golden brown with oil.
4. Assemble the burgers with lettuce, onion, avocado, and enjoy.

**Nutrition values per serving:**
Calories: 776Kcal | Protein: 28.5g | Fat: 30.7g | Carbs: 105.8g

## 105. Quinoa Protein Bars

**Preparation time:** 15 minutes
**Cooking time:** 40 minutes
**Servings:** 10 bars
**Ingredients:**

- ½ cup almonds, chopped
- ½ cup chocolate chips
- ½ cup coconut oil, melted
- ½ cup flaxseed, ground
- ½ cup honey
- ½ tsp. salt
- 1 cup quinoa, dry
- 2 ¼ cup quick oats
- 3 large egg whites

**Directions:**
1. Preheat oven to 325°F.
2. On the bottom of a clean, dry baking sheet, evenly spread oats, quinoa, and almonds. Bake for about 15 minutes or until lightly brown You may want to stir the items in the cookie sheet every few minutes to ensure nothing burns.
3. Remove grains and nuts from the oven and allow to cool completely, but don't turn off the oven.
4. Whisk the egg whites in a bowl and beat the coconut oil and honey into them.
5. Combine flaxseed, chocolate chips, and salt into the cooled grains and nuts, and then pour that mixture into the mixing bowl, coating everything completely.
6. Line your baking sheet with parchment paper and spread the mixture evenly onto it, pressing it into one even layer You may want to shape the sides of the mass, depending on whether or not it reaches the edges of your baking sheet without thinning out too much.
7. Bake for 30 minutes, then remove from the oven. Let cool for one hour before slicing into evenly-shaped bars, then cool completely. Enjoy!

**Nutrition values per bar:**
Calories: 385Kcal | Protein: 8.6g | Fat: 19.8g | Carbs: 45g

## 106. Mediterranean Lamb

**Preparation time:** 10 minutes
**Cooking time:** 35 minutes
**Servings:** 4
**Ingredients:**

- 2 ½ lb. lamb shoulder, cut into chunks
- 1 bay leaf
- 1 cups vegetable stock
- 10 oz. prunes, soaked
- 1 tsp. garlic, minced
- 2 tbsp. honey
- 2 onions, sliced
- 1 tsp. ground cumin
- 1 tsp. ground ginger
- 1 tsp. ground turmeric
- ¼ tsp. cinnamon
- 3 oz. almonds sliced
- Pepper
- Salt

**Directions:**

1. Add all ingredients into the inner pot of the Instant. Pot and stir well.
2. Seal pot with lid and cook on high for 35 minutes.
3. Once done, allow to release pressure naturally. Remove lid. Serve and enjoy!

**Nutrition values per serving:**

Calories: 884Kcal | Protein: 86.6g | Fat: 32g | Carbs: 65.5g

## 107. Coated Cauliflower Head

**Preparation time:** 10 minutes
**Cooking time:** 40 minutes
**Servings:** 2
**Ingredients:**

- 2-lb. cauliflower head
- 3 tbsp. olive oil
- 1 tbsp. butter softened
- 1 tsp. ground coriander
- 1 tsp. salt
- 1 egg, whisked
- 1 tsp. dried cilantro
- 1 tsp. dried oregano
- 1 tsp. Tahini paste

**Directions:**

1. Trim cauliflower head if needed.
2. Preheat oven to 350°F.
3. In the mixing bowl, mix up together olive oil, softened butter, ground coriander, salt, whisked egg, dried cilantro, dried oregano, and tahini paste.
4. Then brush the cauliflower head with this mixture generously and transfer it to the tray.
5. Bake the cauliflower head for 40 minutes.
6. Brush it with the remaining oil mixture every 10 minutes.

**Nutrition values per serving:**

Calories: 393Kcal | Protein: 12.3g | Fat: 30.8g | Carbs: 25.2g

## 108. Artichoke Petals Bites

**Preparation time:** 10 minutes
**Cooking time:** 10 minutes
**Servings:** 2
**Ingredients:**

- 8 oz. artichoke petals, boiled, drained, without salt
- ½ cup almond flour
- 4 oz. parmesan, grated
- 2 tbsp. almond butter, melted

**Directions:**

1. In the mixing bowl, mix up together almond flour and the grated parmesan
2. Preheat the oven to 355°F.
3. Dip the artichoke petals in the almond butter and then coat in the almond flour mixture.
4. Place them in the tray.
5. Transfer the tray to the preheated oven and cook the petals for 10 minutes.
6. Chill the cooked petal bites a little before serving.

**Nutrition values per serving:**

Calories: 508Kcal | Protein: 30.9g | Fat: 34.8g | Carbs: 24.6g

## 109. Stuffed Beef Loin in Sticky Sauce

**Preparation time:** 15 minutes
**Cooking time:** 6 minutes
**Servings:** 4
**Ingredients:**

- 1 tbsp. erythritol
- 1 tbsp. lemon juice
- ½ tsp. tomato sauce
- ¼ tsp. dried rosemary
- 9 oz. beef loin
- 3 oz. celery root, grated
- 3 oz. bacon, sliced
- 1 tbsp. walnuts, chopped
- ¾ tsp. garlic, diced
- 2 tsp. butter
- 1 tbsp. olive oil
- 1 tsp. salt
- ½ cup water

**Directions:**

1. Cut the beef loin into the layer and spread it with the dried rosemary, butter, and salt.
2. Then place over the beef loin: grated celery root, sliced bacon, walnuts, and diced garlic.
3. Roll the beef loin and brush it with olive oil. Secure the meat with the help of the toothpicks.
4. Place it in the tray and add ½ cup water.
5. Cook the meat in the preheated to 365°F oven for 40 minutes.
6. Meanwhile, make the sticky sauce: mix up together erythritol, lemon juice, 4 tbsp. water, and butter.
7. Preheat the mixture until it starts to boil.
8. Then add tomato sauce and whisk it well.

9. Bring the sauce to boil and remove from the heat. When the beef loin is cooked, remove it from the oven and brush it with the cooked sticky sauce very generously. Slice the beef roll and sprinkle with the remaining sauce.

**Nutrition values per serving:**

Calories: 533Kcal | Protein: 59.9g | Fat: 31.5g | Carbs: 2.7g

## 110. Italian Beef Casserole

**Preparation time:** 10 minutes
**Cooking time:** 1 hour 30 minutes
**Servings:** 2
**Ingredients:**

- 1 lb. lean stew beef, cut into chunks
- 3 tsp. paprika
- 4 oz. black olives, sliced
- 7 oz. can crushed tomatoes
- 1 tbsp. tomato puree
- ¼ tsp. garlic powder
- 2 tsp. herb de Provence
- 2 cups beef stock
- 2 tbsp. olive oil

**Directions:**

1. Preheat the oven to 350°F.
2. Heat oil in a pan over medium heat.
3. Add meat to the pan and cook until brown.
4. Add stock, olives, tomatoes, tomato puree, garlic powder, herb de Provence, and paprika Stir well and bring to boil.
5. Transfer the meat mixture to the casserole dish.
6. Cover and cook in preheated oven for 1 ½ hour.
7. Serve and enjoy!

**Nutrition values per serving:**

Calories: 452Kcal | Protein: 16g | Fat: 33.2g | Carbs: 26.8g

## 111. Camembert Mushrooms

**Preparation time:** 8 minutes
**Cooking time:** 5 minutes
**Servings:** 3
**Ingredients:**

- 2 tbsp. butter
- 4 oz. Camembert cheese, diced
- 2 tsp. garlic, minced
- 1 lb. button mushrooms, halved
- black pepper to taste

**Directions:**

1. Place a skillet over medium-high heat. Add the butter and let it melt. Once the butter has melted, add the garlic and sauté until translucent; it should take 3 minutes.
2. Add the mushrooms and cheese and cook for 10 minutes. Season with pepper and serve. Enjoy!

**Nutrition values per serving:**

Calories: 217Kcal | Protein: 12.4g | Fat: 17.3g | Carbs: 5.8g

## 112. Lamb Curry

**Preparation time:** 10 minutes
**Cooking time:** 4 hours
**Servings:** 2
**Ingredients:**

- 2 tbsp. fresh ginger, grated
- 2 garlic cloves, peeled and minced
- 2 tsp. cardamom
- 1 onion, peeled, and chopped
- 6 garlic cloves
- 1 lb. lamb meat, cubed
- 2 tsp. cumin powder
- 1 tsp. gram masala
- ½ tsp. chili powder
- 1 tsp. turmeric
- 2 tsp. coriander
- 1 lb. spinach
- 14 oz. tomatoes, canned

**Directions:**

1. In a slow cooker, mix lamb with tomatoes, spinach, ginger, garlic, onion, cardamom, cloves, cumin, garam masala, chili, turmeric, and coriander.
2. Stir well. Cover and cook on high for 4 hours.
3. Uncover slow cooker, stir the chili, divide into bowls, and serve.

**Nutrition values per serving:**

Calories: 575Kcal | Protein: 74g | Fat: 19.1g | Carbs: 29.3g

## 113. Healthy Baby Carrots

**Preparation time:** 10 minutes
**Cooking time:** 20 minutes
**Servings:** 4
**Ingredients:**

- 1 lb. baby carrots
- 1 tsp. Italian seasoning
- 1 tbsp. balsamic vinegar
- 2 tbsp. olive oil
- ¼ cup vegetable stock
- Pepper
- Salt

**Directions:**

1. Add all ingredients into the inner pot of the Instant. Pot and stir well
2. Seal pot with lid and cook on high for 20 minutes.
3. Once done, allow to release pressure naturally for 5 minutes, then release remaining using quick release. Remove lid.
4. Serve and enjoy!

**Nutrition values per serving:**

Calories: 105Kcal | Protein: 0.8g | Fat: 7.5g | Carbs: 9.6g

## 114. Portobello Mushroom Pizzas with Arugula Salad

**Preparation time:** 35 minutes
**Cooking time:** 45 minutes
**Servings:** 4
**Ingredients:**

- 8 large mushrooms caps portobello
- 2 tbsp. olive oil
- ½ tsp. ground pepper
- ½ cup tomato sauce
- 2 cups spinach
- ½ cup tomato sauce
- 2 cups packed baby spinach
- ½ cup sun-dried tomatoes
- 1 can artichoke hearts
- ½ cup mozzarella cheese
- ¼ cup crumbled feta cheese
- ½ tsp. dried Italian seasoning
- 1 tbsp. lemon juice
- 2 cups baby arugula
- ¼ cup fresh basil leaves

**Directions:**

1. Heat the oven to 400 degrees F.
2. Set a wire rack on a baking sheet with foil. Brush tops with olive oil and place them into the rack for 10 minutes roasting. Flip over and roast them for more 5 minutes.
3. Remove portobellos from the oven and flip them back. Season the sauce inside every cap. Divide spinach, artichokes, feta, mozzarella cheese, and tomatoes among the caps. Spray it with Italian seasoning. Return portobellos to the oven and bake until the cheese is melted and becomes brown for 15 minutes.
4. Mix the remaining ingredients in a bowl and add arugula. Toss them to coat.
5. Garnish the portobello pizzas with basil and serve them immediately.

**Nutrition values per serving:**

Calories: 264kcal | Proteins: 14g | Fats: 13g | Carbs: 25g

## 115. Mediterranean Quinoa with Arugula

**Preparation time:** 15 minutes
**Cooking time:** 3 hours 25 minutes
**Servings:** 6
**Ingredients:**

- ½ cup unsalted vegetable stock
- ½ cup uncooked quinoa
- 1 cup sliced red onions
- 2 garlic cloves
- 1 can chickpeas
- 1 tbsp. olive oil
- ¾ tsp. kosher salt
- 2 tsp. fresh lemon juice
- ½ cup roasted red bell pepper
- 4 cups baby arugula
- 2 oz. feta cheese
- 12 pitted kalamata olives
- 2 tbsp. chopped fresh oregano

**Directions:**

1. Mix garlic, onions, stock, quinoa, chickpeas, olive oil, salt, and onions in a slow cooker. Cover and cook on low heat until the quinoa become soft and the stock is absorbed for 3 to 4 hours.
2. Turn off the slow cooker. Check out the fluffiness of the quinoa mixture by using a fork. Mix the lemon juice and olive oil with salt in it. Add this mixture to the slow cooker. Stir gently to mix and fold in the arugula. Cover and let it stand till the arugula are slightly wilted for almost 10 minutes. Spray every serving smoothly with feta cheese, oregano, and olives.

**Nutrition values per serving:**

Calories: 352kcal | Proteins: 12g | Fats: 13g | Carbs: 46g

## 116. Walnut-Rosemary Crusted Salmon

**Preparation time:** 10 minutes
**Cooking time:** 20 minutes
**Servings:** 4
**Ingredients:**

- 2 tsp. Dijon mustard
- 1 garlic clove

- ¼ tsp. lemon zest
- 1 tsp. lemon juice
- 1 tsp. chopped fresh rosemary
- ½ tsp. honey
- ½ tsp. kosher salt
- ¼ tsp. crushed red pepper
- 3 tbsp. panko breadcrumbs
- 3 tbsp. chopped walnuts
- 1 tsp. olive oil
- 1 pound salmon fillet
- Olive oil spray
- Chopped parsley fresh for garnish

**Directions:**
1. Heat oven to 425 degrees F. Line up a baking sheet along with parchment paper.
2. Mix lemon zest, juice, honey, salt, garlic, mustard, and crushed red bell peppers in a bowl. Mix walnuts, panko, and oil in another bowl.
3. Put salmon on the prepared baking sheet. Spray all the mustard mixture on the fish & spray with the panko mixture. Lightly coat it with cooking spray.
4. Bake till the fish flakes become soft for 8 to 12 minutes depends on the thickness. Spray with parsley & serve it with lemon wedges.

**Nutrition values per serving:**
Calories: 222kcal | Proteins: 24g | Fats: 12g | Carbs: 4g

## 117. Cheesy Artichoke & Spinach Spaghetti Squash

**Preparation time:** 25 minutes
**Cooking time:** 25 minutes
**Servings:** 4
**Ingredients:**
- 2 to 3 pounds spaghetti squash
- 3 tbsp. water
- 1 package baby spinach (455g)
- 1 package frozen artichoke hearts (255g)
- 4 oz. cream cheese
- ½ cup parmesan cheese
- ¼ tsp. salt
- ¼ tsp. ground pepper
- Crushed red pepper for garnish

**Directions:**
1. Put squash in a microwave-safe dish cut side down. Add water to it. Microwave it and increase the heat to a high level till tender for 10 to 15 minutes.
2. Mix spinach & the remaining water in a large skillet on medium heat. Cook till wilted, for almost 3 minutes. Drain out and transfer it to a large bowl.
3. Position rack in the upper third of the oven.
4. Scrape out the squash from the shells in a bowl by using a fork. Put the shells on a baking sheet and mix artichokes, parmesan, cream cheese, pepper, and salt in a squash mixture. Divide it among the squash shells and top it with the remaining ingredients of parmesan cheese. Broil till the cheese become golden brown for almost 3 minutes. Spray with crushed red pepper and basil.

**Nutrition values per serving:**
Calories: 223kcal | Proteins: 10.2g | Fats: 10.9g | Carbs: 23.3g

## 118. Mediterranean Stuffed Chicken Breasts

**Preparation time:** 25 minutes
**Cooking time:** 1 hour
**Servings:** 8
**Ingredients:**
- ½ cup crumbled feta cheese
- ½ cup roasted red bell pepper
- ½ cup fresh chopped spinach
- ¼ cup kalamata olives
- 1 tbsp. chopped fresh basil
- 1 tbsp. chopped leaf parsley
- 2 cloves garlic
- 4 boneless chicken breasts
- ¼ tsp. salt
- ½ tsp. ground pepper
- 1 tbsp. olive oil
- 1 tbsp. lemon juice

**Directions:**
1. Heat the oven to 400 degrees F. mix roasted red peppers, olives, basil, spinach, parsley, and garlic in a bowl.
2. Cut down a horizontal slit by using the thickest portion of every chicken breast to make a pocket using a knife. Stuff every breast pocket with feta mixture. Pack them out with wooden picks. Spray the chicken smoothly with salt and pepper.
3. Heat oil at medium level in an oven skillet. Arrange the stuffed breasts in the pan till golden

for almost 2 minutes. Flip the chicken and transfer the pan to the oven. Bake till a thermometer is inserted in the thickest part of the chicken. Drizzle the chicken smoothly with lemon juice and remove the wooden picks.

**Nutrition values per serving:**

Calories: 179kcal | Proteins: 24.4g | Fats: 7.4g | Carbs: 1.9g

## 119. Charred Shrimp, Pesto & Quinoa Bowls

**Preparation time:** 25 minutes
**Cooking time:** 25 minutes
**Servings:** 4
**Ingredients:**

- 1/3 cup prepared pesto
- 2 tbsp. balsamic vinegar
- 1 tbsp. olive oil
- ½ tsp. salt
- ¼ tsp. ground pepper
- 1-pound large shrimp
- 4 cups arugula
- 2 cups cooked quinoa
- 1 cup cherry tomatoes
- 1 avocado

**Directions:**

1. Mix oil, pepper, salt, pesto, and vinegar in a bowl. Remove mixture to a small bowl and set them aside.
2. Heat a large skillet at medium heat level. Cook the shrimp 4 to 5 minutes, constantly tossing, until they are just cooked through with a little sear. Remove the plate.
3. Add quinoa & arugula to a bowl along with the vinaigrette as well as toss to coat. Split the arugula mixture among four bowls. Top it with avocado, tomatoes, and shrimp. Drizzle every bowl with the reserved pesto mixture.

**Nutrition values per serving:**

Calories: 429kcal | Proteins: 30.9g | Fats: 22g | Carbs: 29.3g

## 120. Sheet-Pan Salmon with Sweet Potatoes & Broccoli

**Preparation time:** 30 minutes
**Cooking time:** 45 minutes
**Servings:** 4
**Ingredients:**

- 3 tbsp. low-fat mayonnaise
- 1 tsp. chili powder
- 2 medium sweet potatoes
- 4 tsp. olive oil
- ½ tsp. salt
- ¼ tsp. ground pepper
- 4 cups broccoli florets
- 1 ¼ pounds salmon fillet
- 2 lemon zest and juice
- ¼ cup crumbled feta cheese
- ½ cup fresh chopped cilantro

**Directions:**

1. Heat the oven to 425 degrees F. line a baking sheet with foil and spray it with cooking spray. Mix chili powder and mayonnaise in a bowl and set them aside.
2. Toss sweet potatoes with salt, pepper, and oil in a bowl. Spray on the prepared baking sheet and roast it for 14 minutes.
3. Toss broccoli with the oil, pepper, and salt in the same bowl. Remove the baking sheet from the oven. Mix the sweet potatoes & move them to the sides of the pan. Arrange salmon at the center of a pan and spray the broccoli on it. Spray mayonnaise over the mixture of salmon. Bake till the sweet potatoes are soft & the salmon flakes for almost 15 minutes. Add lemon juice & zest in the remaining mayonnaise mixture. Divide the salmon into four plates and top it with cheese & cilantro. Drizzle with the mayonnaise sauce and serve it immediately.

**Nutrition values per serving:**

Calories: 504kcal | Proteins: 34g | Fats: 26g | Carbs: 34g

## 121. Mediterranean Ravioli with Artichokes & Olives

**Preparation time:** 15 minutes
**Cooking time:** 15 minutes
**Servings:** 4
**Ingredients:**

- 2 packages frozen spinach
- ½ cup sun-dried tomatoes
- 1 package frozen artichoke hearts
- 1 can cannellini beans
- ¼ cup kalamata olives
- 3 tbsp. pine nuts toasted
- ¼ cup chopped fresh basil

**Directions:**

1. Bring a pot of water to a boil. Cook ravioli as per directions given on the packet. Drain & toss reserved oil and set them aside. Heat the oil in a skillet at medium level.
2. Add beans and artichokes till heated for 3 minutes. Fold it in the cooked ravioli, olives, sun-dried tomatoes, pine nuts & basil.

**Nutrition values per serving:**

Calories: 454kcal | Proteins: 15g | Fats: 19.2g | Carbs: 60.9g

## 122. Slow-Cooker Mediterranean Stew

**Preparation time:** 15 minutes
**Cooking time:** 6 hours 45 minutes
**Servings:** 6
**Ingredients:**

- 2 cans roasted diced tomatoes
- 3 cups vegetable broth
- 1 cup chopped onions
- ¾ cup chopped carrot
- 4 cloves garlic
- 1 tsp. dried oregano
- ¾ tsp. salt
- ½ tsp. crushed red pepper
- ¼ tsp. ground pepper
- 1 can chickpeas
- 1 bunch lacinato kale
- 1 tbsp. lemon juice
- 2 tbsp. olive oil
- Fresh basil leaves
- 6 lemon wedges

**Directions:**

1. Mix tomatoes, carrot, oregano, salt, garlic, onion, broth, pepper, red pepper in a slow cooker. Cover it and cook it for almost 6 hours.
2. Measure cooking liquid from the slow cooker and add in another bowl. Add chickpeas and mash them by using a fork till smooth.
3. Add the kale, lemon juice, mashed chickpeas, & whole chickpeas to the mixture in the slow cooker. Mix to combine. Cover it and cook it on low heat till the kale is soft, around 30 minutes. Ladle the stew smoothly in 6 bowls and drizzle them with oil.

**Nutrition values per serving:**

Calories: 191kcal | Proteins: 5.7g | Fats: 7.8g | Carbs: 23g

## 123. Greek Cauliflower Rice Bowls with Grilled Chicken

**Preparation time:** 30 minutes
**Cooking time:** 30 minutes
**Servings:** 4
**Ingredients:**

- 6 tbsp. olive oil
- 4 cups cauliflower rice
- 1/3 cup red onion chopped
- ¾ tsp. salt
- ½ cup chopped fresh dill
- 1 pound chicken breasts
- ½ tsp. ground pepper
- 3 tbsp. lemon juice
- 1 tsp. dried oregano
- 1 cup cherry tomatoes
- 1 cup chopped cucumber
- 2 tbsp. chopped kalamata olives
- 2 tbsp. crumbled feta cheese
- 4 lemon wedges

**Directions:**

1. Heat the grill on medium. Heat oil in a skillet on medium heat. Add onion, cauliflower, and salt. Cook till the cauliflower becomes tender for almost 5 minutes. Remove it from the heat and stir it in a dill.
2. Rub oil on all the chicken. Spray with salt, pepper. Grill it till the thermometer inserted into the thickest part of the breast reads 165 degrees F. slice it crosswise. Mix remaining oil, oregano, lemon juice, pepper, and salt in a bowl.
3. Divide cauliflower rice into 4 bowls. Top it with chicken, cucumber, tomatoes, olives & feta. Sprinkle it with the remaining 1/4 cup dill. Drizzle it with vinaigrette. Serve it with lemon wedges.

**Nutrition values per serving:**

Calories: 411kcal | Proteins: 29g | Fats: 27.5g | Carbs: 9.5g

## 124. Prosciutto Pizza with Corn & Arugula

**Preparation time:** 20 minutes
**Cooking time:** 20 minutes
**Servings:** 4

**Ingredients:**
- 1 pound pizza dough
- 2 tbsp. olive oil
- 1 garlic clove
- 1 cup shredded mozzarella cheese
- 1 cup fresh corn kernels
- 1 -ounce sliced prosciutto
- 1 ½ cups arugula
- ½ cup fresh torn basil
- ¼ tsp. ground pepper

**Directions:**
1. Heat grill to medium heat.
2. Roll dough on a floured surface. Transfer it to a lightly floured large baking sheet. Mix garlic and oil in a bowl. Bring the dough, cheese, corn, garlic oil, and prosciutto to the grill.
3. Oil the grill racks. Transfer it to the crust of the grill. Grill the dough till puffed & lightly browned for almost 2 minutes.
4. Flip the crust and spread the garlic oil on it. Top it with cheese, corn & prosciutto. Grill till the cheese melts and the crust is browned from the bottom. Return the pizza to the baking sheet.
5. Top it with pizza arugula, basil, and pepper.

**Nutrition values per serving:**
Calories: 436kcal | Proteins: 18.3g | Fats: 19.9g | Carbs: 53.1g

## 125. Vegan Mediterranean Lentil Soup

**Preparation time:** 20 minutes
**Cooking time:** 1 hour
**Servings:** 6
**Ingredients:**
- 2 tbsp. olive oil
- 1 ½ cup chopped yellow onions
- 1 cup chopped carrots
- 3 garlic cloves
- 2 tbsp. tomato paste
- 4 cups vegetable broth
- 1 cup water
- 1 can cannellini beans
- 1 cup dry lentils
- ½ cup sun-dried tomatoes
- ¾ tsp. salt
- ½ tsp. ground pepper
- 1 tbsp. chopped fresh dill
- 1 ½ tsp. red-wine vinegar

**Directions:**
1. Heat oil in a heavy pot on medium heat. Add carrots and onions. Cook till softened for 4 minutes. Add garlic and cook till fragrant for almost 1 min. Add tomato paste and cook till the mixture is smoothly coated for 1 min.
2. Stir in water, broth, lentils, tomatoes, pepper, salt, and cannellini beans. Bring to a boil on medium heat. Cover and simmer till the lentils become soft for 35 minutes.
3. Remove it from the heat & stir in dill and vinegar. Garnish it with additional dill and serve it.

**Nutrition values per serving:**
Calories: 272kcal | Proteins: 13g | Fats: 7g | Carbs: 42g

## 126. Eggplant & Parmesan

**Preparation time:** 25 minutes
**Cooking time:** 45 minutes
**Servings:** 6
**Ingredients:**
- olive oil
- 2 large eggs
- 2 tbsp. water
- 1 cup panko breadcrumbs
- ¾ cup parmesan cheese
- 1 tsp. Italian seasoning
- 2 medium eggplants
- ½ tsp. salt
- ½ tsp. ground pepper
- 1 jar tomato sauce
- ¼ cup fresh basil leaves
- 2 garlic cloves
- ½ tsp. crushed red pepper
- 1 cup shredded mozzarella cheese

**Directions:**
1. Place racks in the middle and lower thirds of an oven. Heat oven to 400 degrees F. coat two baking sheets & baking dish with cooking spray.
2. Mix water & eggs in a bowl. Mix parmesan, Italian seasonings, and breadcrumbs in a dish. Dig eggplant in the egg mixture. Coat with the breadcrumb mixture.
3. Arrange the eggplant in a single layer on the prepared baking sheets. Spray both sides of the eggplant with cooking spray.

4. Bake, toss the eggplant, & swap the pans between racks halfway until the eggplant is softly browned for almost 30 minutes. Season it with salt & pepper.
5. Mix tomato sauce, garlic, basil, and crushed red pepper in a bowl. Spread the sauce in the prepared dish. Arrange half the eggplant slices over the sauce.
6. Spoon sauce on the eggplant and sprinkle with parmesan and mozzarella cheese. Bake till the sauce is bubbling and the top is golden for 25 minutes. Let it cool for 5 minutes. Spray it with more basil before serving.

**Nutrition values per serving:**
Calories: 241kcal | Proteins: 14g | Fats: 9g | Carbs: 28g

## 127. B.B.Q. Shrimp with Garlicky Kale & Parmesan-Herb Couscous

**Preparation time:** 20 minutes
**Cooking time:** 20 minutes
**Servings:** 4
**Ingredients:**
- 1 cup chicken broth
- ¼ tsp. poultry seasoning
- 2/3 cup whole white couscous
- 1/3 cup parmesan cheese
- 1 tbsp. butter
- 3 tbsp. olive oil
- 8 cups chopped kale
- ¼ cup water
- 1 large garlic clove
- ¼ tsp. crushed red pepper
- ¼ tsp. salt
- 1-pound raw shrimp
- ¼ cup B.B.Q. sauce

**Directions:**
1. Mix poultry and broth seasoning in a saucepan and cook on medium heat.
2. Bring to a boil and stir in couscous. Remove it from the heat, cover it and let it stand for 5 minutes. Fluff it with a fork & stir butter and parmesan. Cover to keep warm.
3. Heat oil in a large skillet on medium heat. Add kale & cook till bright green for 2 minutes. Add water, cover, and cook till the kale is tender for almost 3 minutes. Reduce heat to medium-low. Make a well at the kale center and add oil, red pepper, garlic, and oil into the kale. Season it with salt. Transfer to a bowl & cover it to keep warm.
4. Add oil and shrimp to the pan. Cook till the shrimp are pink & curled. Remove it from the heat and mix in B.B.Q. Sauce. Serve immediately.

**Nutrition values per serving:**
Calories: 414kcal | Proteins: 32.2g | Fats: 16.9g | Carbs: 36.4g

## 128. Shakshuka with Spinach, Chard & Feta

**Preparation time:** 30 minutes
**Cooking time:** 30 minutes
**Servings:** 6
**Ingredients:**
- 1/3 cup olive oil
- 1 large onion
- 12 oz. chopped chard, stemmed
- 12 oz. mature spinach
- ½ cup dry white wine
- 1 small jalapeno
- 2 medium garlic cloves
- ¼ tsp. kosher salt
- ¼ tsp. ground pepper
- ½ cup chicken broth low sodium
- 6 large eggs
- 2 tbsp. unsalted butter
- ½ cup crumbled feta cheese

**Directions:**
1. Heat oil in a skillet on medium heat. Add onion and cook till soft and translucent but not browned for almost 8 minutes. Add spinach and chard and cook till wilted for almost 5 minutes. Add jalapeno, salt, pepper, wine, and garlic and cook till the wine is absorbed and the garlic softens for 2 to 4 minutes.
2. Add butter and broth to it. Cook till the butter is melted, and some of the liquid is absorbed for almost 2 minutes.
3. Split eggs on the veggies and cover them. Cook over medium heat till the whites are set for 5 minutes. Remove from the heat and spray with cheese. Cover it and let it stand for 2 minutes before serving.

**Nutrition values per serving:**
Calories: 296kcal | Proteins: 10.7g | Fats: 23.4g | Carbs: 8.5g

## 129. One-Skillet Salmon with Fennel & Sun-Dried Tomato Couscous

**Preparation time:** 30 minutes
**Cooking time:** 40 minutes
**Servings:** 4
**Ingredients:**

- 1 lemon
- 1 ¼ pounds salmon
- ¼ tsp. salt
- ¼ tsp. ground pepper
- 4 tbsp. sun-dried tomato paste
- 2 tbsp. olive oil
- 2 medium fennel bulbs
- 1 cup Israeli couscous
- 3 scallions
- 1 ½ cups chicken broth low sodium
- ¼ cup green olives
- 2 tbsp. toasted pine nuts
- 2 garlic cloves

**Directions:**

1. Cut the lemon zest into 8 slices. Season salmon with salt and pepper. Spread pesto on every piece.
2. Heat oil in a skillet on medium-high heat. Add half the fennel, cook till brown from the bottom for 3 minutes. Transfer it to a plate.
3. Reduce heat to medium and repeat it with the remaining oil and fennel.
4. Transfer to the plate. Add couscous and scallions to the pan and cook till the couscous is toasted for 2 minutes. Stir in broth, pine nuts, lemon zest, pesto, and garlic. Nestle the salmon & fennel into the couscous. Top it with salmon and lemon slices. Lower the heat to low and cook till the salmon is cooked through & the couscous is soft for 13 minutes. Garnish it with fennel fronds.

**Nutrition values per serving:**
Calories: 543kcal | Proteins: 38.3g | Fats: 24.1g | Carbs: 46g

## 130. Spinach & Chicken Skillet Pasta with Parmesan & Lemon

**Preparation time:** 25 minutes
**Cooking time:** 25 minutes
**Servings:** 4
**Ingredients:**

- 8 oz. penne pasta gluten-free
- 2 tbsp. olive oil
- 1 pound chicken breasts
- ½ tsp. salt
- ¼ tsp. ground pepper
- 4 garlic cloves
- ½ cup dry white wine
- 1 lemon juice and zest
- 10 cups chopped fresh spinach
- 4 tbsp. grated parmesan cheese

**Directions:**

1. Cook pasta according to the package directions. Drain and set them aside.
2. Heat oil in a high skillet on medium heat. Add salt, pepper, chicken, and cook till just cooked for 7 minutes.
3. Add garlic and cook till fragrant for 1 min. Stir in wine, zest, and lemon juice; bring to a boil.
4. Would you please remove it from the heat?
5. Stir in spinach and the cooked pasta. Cover and let them stand till the spinach are just wilted. Divide among 4 plates and top with parmesan.

**Nutrition values per serving:**
Calories: 335kcal | Proteins: 28.7g | Fats: 12.3g | Carbs: 24.9g

## 131. Quinoa, Avocado & Chickpea Salad over Mixed Greens

**Preparation time:** 25 minutes
**Cooking time:** 15 minutes
**Servings:** 2
**Ingredients:**

- 2/3 cup water
- 1/3 cup quinoa
- ¼ tsp. kosher salt
- 1 garlic clove
- 2 tsp. lemon zest
- 3 tbsp. lemon juice
- 3 tbsp. olive oil
- ¼ tsp. ground pepper
- 1 cup canned chickpeas
- 1 medium carrot, shredded
- ½ avocado
- 1 package mixed greens & spinach (5 oz.)

**Directions:**

1. In a saucepan, bring water to a boil and stir in quinoa. Reduce heat to low, cover, and boil it until all the liquid is absorbed for 15 minutes. Use a fork to fluff and separate the grains and let them cool for 5 minutes.
2. On a cutting board, sprinkle salt over garlic. Mash the garlic by using a spoon till paste forms. Scrape in a medium bowl.
3. Mix lemon zest, juice, pepper, and oil. Transfer the dressing to a bowl and set them aside.
4. Add carrot, avocado, and chickpeas to the bowl and gently toss them. Let them stand for 4 minutes to allow flavors to blend. Add the quinoa and place greens in a bowl. Toss with the reserved dressing and divide the greens among plates. Top it with a mixture of quinoa.

**Nutrition values per serving:**
Calories: 501kcal | Proteins: 12g | Fats: 31.5g | Carbs: 47.3g

## 132. Sheet-Pan Mediterranean Chicken, Brussels Sprouts & Gnocchi

**Preparation time:** 20 minutes
**Cooking time:** 40 minutes
**Servings:** 4
**Ingredients:**

- 4 tbsp. olive oil
- 2 tbsp. chopped fresh oregano
- 2 large garlic cloves
- ½ tsp. ground pepper
- ¼ tsp. salt
- 1 pound brussels sprouts
- 1 package shelf-stable gnocchi
- 1 cup sliced red onion
- 4 boneless chicken thighs
- 1 cup cherry tomatoes
- 1 tbsp. red-wine vinegar

**Directions:**

1. Heat the oven to 450 degrees F. Mix oil, oregano, pepper, garlic, and salt in a bowl. Add Brussel sprouts, onion, and gnocchi. Toss to coat. Spread it on a baking sheet.
2. Mix oil, garlic, oregano, pepper, and salt in a bowl. Add chicken into it and toss to coat. Nestle the chicken in the veggie mixture. Roast it for 10 minutes.
3. Remove it from the oven and add tomatoes into it. Mix it well. Continue roasting till the brussels sprouts are softened. Chicken is cooked thoroughly for almost 10 minutes. Stir vinegar and the remaining oil into the veggie mixture.

**Nutrition values per serving:**
Calories: 604kcal | Proteins: 39.1g | Fats: 23.9g | Carbs: 60.6g

## 133. Caprese Stuffed Portobello Mushrooms

**Preparation time:** 25 minutes
**Cooking time:** 40 minutes
**Servings:** 4
**Ingredients:**

- 3 tbsp. olive oil
- 1 medium c garlic love
- ½ tsp. salt
- ½ tsp. ground pepper
- 4 mushrooms portobello
- 1 cup cherry tomatoes
- ½ cup fresh mozzarella pearls
- ½ cup fresh basil
- 2 tsp. balsamic vinegar

**Directions:**

1. Heat the oven to 400 degrees F.
2. Mix oil, salt, pepper, garlic in a bowl. Put it on a baking sheet and bake till the mushrooms are soft for almost 10 minutes using a silicon brush.
3. Mix mozzarella, salt, pepper, oil, tomatoes, and basil together in a bowl. Remove from the oven after softening of mushrooms. Fill it with tomato mixture.
4. Bake till the cheese is completely melted & the tomatoes have become wilted for almost 15 minutes more. Drizzle every mushroom with vinegar and serve immediately.

**Nutrition values per serving:**
Calories: 186kcal | Proteins: 6.3g | Fats: 16g | Carbs: 6.3g

## 134. Sweet & Spicy Roasted Salmon with Wild Rice Pilaf

**Preparation time:** 15 minutes
**Cooking time:** 30 minutes
**Servings:** 4
**Ingredients:**

- 5 salmon fillets
- 2 tbsp. balsamic vinegar

- 1 tbsp. honey
- ¼ tsp. salt
- 1/8 tsp. ground pepper
- 1 cup chopped bell pepper
- 1 small jalapeno
- 2 scallions
- ¼ cup chopped parsley
- 2 2/3 cups wild rice pilaf

**Directions:**
1. Heat the oven to 425 degrees F after thawing frozen salmon. Line a baking sheet with parchment paper. Put the salmon in the prepared pan.
2. Mix vinegar and honey in a bowl. Drizzle over it and spray salt and pepper on it.
3. Roast the salmon till the thickest part flakes for almost 15 minutes. Drizzle it with the remaining vinegar mixture.
4. Coat a skillet with cooking spray on medium heat. Add bell pepper and jalapeno. Cook till tender for almost 5 minutes. Remove from the heat. Mix in scallion greens.
5. Top four of the salmon fillets with the pepper mixture and parsley.

**Nutrition values per serving:**
Calories: 339kcal | Proteins: 29.6g | Fats: 5.3g | Carbs: 42.5g

## 135. Zucchini Lasagna Rolls with Smoked Mozzarella

**Preparation time:** 30 minutes
**Cooking time:** 1 hour
**Servings:** 4
**Ingredients:**
- 2 large zucchini
- 2 tsp. olive oil
- ½ tsp. ground pepper
- ¼ tsp. salt
- 8 tbsp. shredded smoked mozzarella cheese - 3 tbsp. parmesan cheese grated
- 1 large egg
- 1 1/3 cups ricotta
- 1 package frozen spinach (10 oz.)
- 1 clove garlic
- ¾ cup marinara sauce
- 2 tbsp. chopped fresh basil

**Directions:**
1. Put racks in the upper thirds of the oven and heat it to 425 degrees F.
2. Slice zucchini lengthwise to obtain 24 strips.
3. Toss the zucchini, salt, oil, and pepper in a bowl. Arrange the zucchini in single layers on the already prepared pans.
4. Bake the zucchini, whirling once, till tender for almost 10 minutes total.
5. Mix mozzarella and parmesan in a bowl. Mix ricotta, garlic, spinach, egg, pepper, and salt in a bowl.
6. Spread marinara in a baking dish and put ricotta mixture at the bottom of the strip of zucchini. Roll it in a baking dish. Repeat it with the remaining zucchini. Fill it and top it with marinara sauce and spray with the reserved cheese mixture.
7. Bake it till bubbly and browned on top for almost 20 minutes. Let it stand for 4 minutes. Spray with basil before serving.

**Nutrition values per serving:**
Calories: 315kcal | Proteins: 22.2g | Fats: 18.6g | Carbs: 16.8g

## 136. Herby Mediterranean Tilapia with Wilted Greens & Mushrooms

**Preparation time:** 25 minutes
**Cooking time:** 25 minutes
**Servings:** 4
**Ingredients:**
- 3 tbsp. olive oil
- ½ large sweet onion
- 3 cups cremini mushrooms
- 2 garlic cloves
- 4 cups chopped kale
- 1 medium tomato
- 2 tsp. Mediterranean herbs mix
- 1 tbsp. lemon juice
- ½ tsp. salt
- ½ tsp. ground pepper
- 4-ounce tilapia fillets
- Fresh parsley for garnish

**Directions:**
1. Heat oil in a saucepan on medium heat. Add the onion in it and cook till translucent for 4 minutes. Add garlic and mushrooms and cook till

mushrooms release their piqued and begin to brown.
2. Add tomato, kale, and herb mix and cook till the kale is wilted. Mushrooms become soft for 7 minutes. Mix in lemon juice, salt, and pepper.
3. Remove from the heat, cover it, and keep warm. Sprinkle fish with herb mix, salt, pepper, oil in a saucepan on medium heat. Add the fish and cook till the flesh is opaque for 3 minutes depends on the thickness.
4. Transfer the fish to a serving plate. Top it with veggies and parsley.

**Nutrition values per serving:**
Calories: 214kcal | Proteins: 18g | Fats: 11g | Carbs: 11g

## 137. Chicken with Tomato-Balsamic Pan Sauce

**Preparation time:** 35 minutes
**Cooking time:** 35 minutes
**Servings:** 4
**Ingredients:**
- 2 8-oz. chicken breasts
- ½ tsp. salt
- ½ tsp. ground pepper
- ¼ cup whole wheat flour
- 3 tbsp. olive oil
- ½ cup cherry tomatoes
- 2 tbsp. sliced shallot
- ¼ cup balsamic vinegar
- 1 cup chicken broth
- 1 tbsp. minced garlic
- 1 tbsp. fennel seeds
- 1 tbsp. butter

**Directions:**
1. Remove and reserve chicken tenders for use. Slice every breast in half to get 4 pieces. Put on a cutting board and cover with a large piece of plastic wrap. Sprinkle with salt and pepper. Place flour in a shallow bowl and coat cutlets from both sides.
2. Heat oil in a skillet on medium heat. Add 2 pieces of chicken and cook till browned and cooked through for 3 minutes per side. Transfer it to a large serving plate and keep it warm by using foil. Add tomatoes, shallot, and oil into the pan. Cook till softened for 2 minutes. Add vinegar and bring to simmer. Cook browned bits at the bottom of the pan till the vinegar is reduced by half for almost 45 seconds. Add garlic, broth, pepper, and salt and cook until the sauce is reduced by half for 7 minutes. Remove from heat and mix it well in butter.

**Nutrition values per serving:**
Calories: 294kcal | Proteins: 25.4g | Fats: 16.7g | Carbs: 9.5g

## 138. Healthy Lemon Bars

**Preparation time:** 15 minutes
**Cooking time:** 25 minutes
**Servings:** 4
**Ingredients:**
For crust
- 1/4 cup butter
- ¼ cup pure maple syrup
- ¼ tsp. almond extract
- 1 1/2 cups packed almond flour
- 2 tbsp. coconut flour
- 1/4 tsp. salt

For filling
- Zest from 1 lemon
- 2/3 cup freshly squeezed lemon juice
- ½ cup pure maple syrup
- 4 large eggs
- 1 tbsp. coconut flour

To garnish
- Lemon zest
- Powdered sugar (sifted)

**Directions:**
1. Heat the oven to 350 degrees F. Line a baking sheet on parchment paper.
2. Make the crust and mix the almond flour, salt, and coconut flour in it. Mix in the butter, almond extract, and maple syrup till a dough form. Press dough properly and smoothly in a prepared pan and bake for 15 minutes.
3. Make filling after making crust bakes in a bowl. Mix lemon juices, zest, eggs, maple syrup, and coconut flour. Blend them well. Pour filling over crust after baking is done. Do it fast, and don't let them cool down. Reduce the temperature to 325 degrees F. put bars in an oven and bake the bars for 20 minutes till filling is set. Cool on a wire rack and refrigerate it for 4 hours. Once bars become firm, it's ready to serve.

**Nutrition values per serving:**
Calories: 189kcal | Proteins: 4.9g | Fats: 11.5g | Carbs: 18.9g

## 139. Roasted Pistachio-Crusted Salmon with Broccoli

**Preparation time:** 30 minutes
**Cooking time:** 45 minutes
**Servings:** 4
**Ingredients:**

- 8 cups broccoli florets
- 2 garlic cloves
- 3 tbsp. olive oil
- ¾ tsp. salt
- ½ tsp. ground pepper
- ½ cup salted pistachios
- 2 tbsp. chopped fresh chives
- 1 medium lemon zest
- 4 tsp. mayonnaise
- 1 ¼ pound salmon fillet

**Directions:**

1. Heat oven to 425 degrees F. coat a baking sheet with cooking spray. Combine broccoli, oil, salt, garlic, and pepper on the baking sheet. Roast till for 5 minutes.
2. Mix chives, lemon zest, oil, pistachios, pepper, and salt in a bowl. Sprinkle mayonnaise on every salmon part and top it with the pistachio's mixture.
3. Move the broccoli to one side of the baking sheet and put salmon on the space. Roast it till salmon is opaque in the center and the broccoli is soft for 10 to 15 minutes, depending on the thickness.

**Nutrition values per serving:**
Calories: 424kcal | Proteins: 36g | Fats: 26.7g | Carbs: 12.3g

# CHAPTER 14

# Snacks

## 140. Everything-Bagel Crispy Chickpeas

**Preparation time:** 10 minutes
**Cooking time:** 50 minutes
**Servings:** 6
**Ingredients:**

- 2 cans chickpeas
- 3 tbsp. olive oil
- 2 tbsp. bagel seasoning

**Directions:**

1. Put a rack in the top third part of the oven. Put a large baking sheet on the rack. Heat the oven to 400 degrees F.
2. Line a baking sheet along with paper towels. Sprinkle chickpeas on the paper towel and rub it with more to discard skins.
3. Toss the chickpeas & oil in a bowl. Sprinkle it in a smooth layer on the hot layer of the baking sheet. Roast till crispy and golden brown for almost 30 minutes.
4. Grind everything bagel seasoning in a spice grinder. When the chickpeas are ready, spray the hot chickpeas with the seasoning and toss to coat. Let them cool for 10 minutes before serving.

**Nutrition values per serving:**
Calories: 220kcal | Proteins: 8.5g | Fats: 8.4g | Carbs: 25.4g

## 141. Kale Chips

**Preparation time:** 15 minutes
**Cooking time:** 15 minutes
**Servings:** 2
**Ingredients:**

- Cooking spray
- 6 cups kale leaves
- 1 tbsp. olive oil
- 1 ½ tsp. soy sauce
- 1/8 tsp. salt
- ½ tsp. white sesame seeds
- ¼ tsp. ground cumin

**Directions:**

1. Coat the air fryer basket along with cooking spray.
2. Toss kale with oil, salt, and soy sauce in a bowl. Rub the leaves together so they are properly coated.
3. Put the kale mix in the already prepared basket. Coat the leaves along with cooking spray. Cook at 375 degrees F till crispy for almost 10 minutes. Shake the basket and mix the leaves every 3 minutes. Remove from the basket quickly and spray with sesame seeds & cumin.

**Nutrition values per serving:**
Calories: 140kcal | Proteins: 4.4g | Fats: 9.4g | Carbs: 12.8g

## 142. Peanut Butter Energy Balls

**Preparation time:** 20 minutes
**Cooking time:** 20 minutes
**Servings:** 17
**Ingredients:**

- 2 cups rolled oats
- 1 cup natural peanut butter
- ½ cup honey
- ¼ cups mini chocolate chips
- ¼ cup unsweetened shredded coconut

**Directions:**

1. Mix peanut butter, oats, chocolate chips, honey, & coconut in a bowl. Stir it properly and well.
2. Measure all the remaining ingredients and make a mixture of them that is ball shaped. Store in a container (airtight) in the refrigerator for 5 days.

**Nutrition values per serving:**
Calories: 174kcal | Proteins: 4.4g | Fats: 9.2g | Carbs: 18.2g

## 143. Avocado Hummus

**Preparation time:** 10 minutes
**Cooking time:** 10 minutes
**Servings:** 10
**Ingredients:**

- 1 can chickpeas
- 1 ripe avocado
- 1 cup fresh cilantro
- ¼ cup tahini
- ¼ cup olive oil
- ¼ cup lemon juice
- 1 garlic clove
- 1 tsp. ground cumin
- ½ tsp. salt

**Directions:**

1. Drain chickpeas after washing and reserve them in the liquid.
2. Transfer these things to a blender.
3. Add garlic, oil, tahini, lemon juice, avocado, cilantro, salt, and cumin and blend it till smooth. Serve with veggies.

**Nutrition values per serving:**
Calories: 156kcal | Proteins: 3.3g | Fats: 12.4g | Carbs: 9.5g

## 144. Fig & Honey Yogurt

**Preparation time:** 5 minutes
**Cooking time:** 0 minutes
**Servings:** 1
**Ingredients:**

- 2/3 cup plain yogurt
- 1 dried fig
- 2 tsp. honey

**Directions:**

1. Put the yogurt in a bowl & top it with honey & figs.

**Nutrition values per serving:**
Calories: 208kcal | Proteins: 9g | Fats: 2.8g | Carbs: 39g

## 145. Cheesy Vegan Brussels Sprout Chips

**Preparation time:** 20 minutes
**Cooking time:** 20 minutes
**Servings:** 4
**Ingredients:**

- 15 brussels sprouts
- 1 tbsp. olive oil
- 1 tsp. nutritional yeast
- ¼ tsp. ground pepper
- 1/8 tsp. salt

**Directions:**

1. Heat an oven to 400 degrees F.
2. Remove outer leaves from Brussel sprouts and make 4 cups. Put them in a bowl and add oil, pepper, salt, yeast.
3. Gently massage the leaves properly till coated.
4. Roast till the leaves get crispy and browned after spreading a single layer on a baking sheet for 10 minutes.

**Nutrition values per serving:**
Calories: 45kcal | Proteins: 1.2g | Fats: 3.6g | Carbs: 2.5g

## 146. Cinnamon-Sugar Roasted Chickpeas

**Preparation time:** 5 minutes
**Cooking time:** 55 minutes
**Servings:** 4
**Ingredients:**

- 1 can chickpeas
- 1 tbsp. sugar
- 1 tsp. ground cinnamon
- 1/8 tsp. ground pepper
- 1 tbsp. avocado oil

**Directions:**

1. Put rack back to the upper third part of the oven. Heat the oven to 450 degrees F.
2. Blot chickpeas to dry out. Sprinkle it on a baking sheet.
3. Bake it for 10 minutes and mix pepper, cinnamon, and sugar into it.
4. Transfer the chickpeas to a bowl and oil them with a sugar-cinnamon mixture. Please return to the baking sheet and bake it again for mixing till browned & crunchy for 20 minutes. Let them cool on the baking sheet for 14 minutes.

**Nutrition values per serving:**
Calories: 125kcal | Proteins: 4.7g | Fats: 4.5g | Carbs: 16.4g

## 147. Carrot Cake Energy Bites

**Preparation time:** 15 minutes
**Cooking time:** 15 minutes
**Servings:** 22

**Ingredients:**
- 1 cup pitted dates
- ½ cup rolled oats
- ¼ cup chopped pecans
- ¼ cup chia seeds
- 2 medium carrots
- 1 tsp. vanilla extract
- ¾ tsp. ground cinnamon
- ½ tsp. ground ginger
- ¼ tsp. ground turmeric
- ¼ tsp. salt
- 1 pinch ground pepper

**Directions:**
1. Mix oats, pecans, dates, and chia seeds in a blender till chopped and well mixed.
2. Add carrots, ginger, turmeric, vanilla, cinnamon, salt, and pepper. Process it till all the ingredients are properly chopped as well as a paste starts to form.
3. Roll the mixture in balls by using a scant.

**Nutrition values per serving:**
Calories: 48kcal | Proteins: 0.9g | Fats: 1.7g | Carbs: 8.2g

## 148. Cucumber Hummus Sandwiches

**Preparation time:** 5 minutes
**Cooking time:** 5 minutes
**Servings:** 1
**Ingredients:**
- 5 tsp. hummus
- 10 slices cucumber

**Directions:**
1. Sprinkle hummus on a slice of a cucumber and top it with a second cucumber on it as a slice.
2. Repeat the process to make 5 to 6 sandwiches.

**Nutrition values per serving:**
Calories: 47kcal | Proteins: 2g | Fats: 2g | Carbs: 5g

## 149. White Bean & Avocado Toast

**Preparation time:** 5 minutes
**Cooking time:** 5 minutes
**Servings:** 1
**Ingredients:**
- 1 slice whole-wheat bread
- ¼ mashed avocado
- ½ cup canned white beans
- Kosher salt
- Ground pepper
- 1 pinch crushed red pepper

**Directions:**
1. Top the toast with white beans & mashed avocado.
2. Season it with salt, crushed red pepper, and pepper.

**Nutrition values per serving:**
Calories: 230kcal | Proteins: 11.5g | Fats: 8.8g | Carbs: 34.7g

## 150. Tomato-Basil Skewers

**Preparation time:** 10 minutes
**Cooking time:** 10 minutes
**Servings:** 16
**Ingredients:**
- 16 small fresh mozzarella balls
- 16 basil leaves
- 16 cherry tomatoes
- Olive oil
- Salt & pepper to taste

**Directions:**
1. Yarn mozzarella, basil & tomatoes on a small skewer.
2. Drizzle it with oil & sprinkle it with pepper & salt.

**Nutrition values per serving:**
Calories: 46kcal | Proteins: 2.8g | Fats: 3.3g | Carbs: 1g

## 151. Garlic Hummus

**Preparation time:** 10 minutes
**Cooking time:** 10 minutes
**Servings:** 8
**Ingredients:**
- 1 can chickpeas
- ¼ cup tahini
- ¼ cup olive oil
- ¼ cup lemon juice
- 1 garlic clove
- 1 tsp. ground cumin
- ½ tsp. chili powder
- ½ tsp. salt

**Directions:**
1. Drain out chickpeas and reserve them in the liquid.

2. Transfer them to a blender and add oil, tahini, cumin, garlic, salt, lemon juice, and chili powder. Puree till becomes smooth for 3 minutes.

**Nutrition values per serving:**

Calories: 155kcal | Proteins: 3.7g | Fats: 11.9g | Carbs: 9.7g

## 152. Savory Date & Pistachio Bites

**Preparation time:** 10 minutes
**Cooking time:** 10 minutes
**Servings:** 32 bites
**Ingredients:**

- 2 cups whole dates
- 1 cup unsalted pistachios
- 1 cup golden raisins
- 1 tsp. ground fennel seeds
- ¼ tsp. ground pepper

**Directions:**

1. Mix dates, raisins, fennel, pistachios, and pepper in a food processor. Process till finely and well chopped. Make them into 32 balls by using 1 tbsp. each.

**Nutrition values per bite:**

Calories: 68kcal | Proteins: 1.1g | Fats: 1.8g | Carbs: 13.4g

## 153. Roasted Buffalo Chickpeas

**Preparation time:** 5 minutes
**Cooking time:** 35 minutes
**Servings:** 4
**Ingredients:**

- 1 tbsp. white vinegar
- ½ tsp. cayenne pepper
- ¼ tsp. salt
- 1 can chickpeas

**Directions:**

1. Put the rack in the upper third part of an oven and heat to 400 degrees F.
2. Mix vinegar, salt, and cayenne in a bowl. Pat chickpeas dry and toss along with vinegar mixture.
3. Sprinkle on a baking sheet and roast the chickpeas till browned and crunchy for 30 minutes. Let them cool for 30 more minutes till the chickpeas become well crisp.

**Nutrition values per serving:**

Calories: 109kcal | Proteins: 5.8g | Fats: 0.9g | Carbs: 17.6g

## 154. Pistachio & Peach Toast

**Preparation time:** 5 minutes
**Cooking time:** 5 minutes
**Servings:** 1
**Ingredients:**

- 1 tbsp. ricotta cheese
- 1 tsp. honey
- 1/8 tsp. cinnamon
- 1 slice whole-wheat bread
- ½ medium peach
- 1 tbsp. chopped pistachios

**Directions:**

1. Mix ricotta, honey & cinnamon in a bowl.
2. Sprinkle the ricotta mixture on toast and top it with peach 7 pistachios.
3. Drizzle it with honey.

**Nutrition values per serving:**

Calories: 193kcal | Proteins: 8.2g | Fats: 6g | Carbs: 29g

## 155. Grilled Flatbread with Burrata Cheese

**Preparation time:** 15 minutes
**Cooking time:** 20 minutes
**Servings:** 6
**Ingredients:**

Tomato skewers

- 18 oz. cherry tomatoes
- Olive oil
- Pepper & salt
- 4 skewers for grilling

Flatbread

- 1 lb. pizza dough
- Flour for dusting
- ¾ cup olive oil
- 8 oz. burrata cheese
- 8 oz. parmesan cheese
- 2 tbsp. fresh basil

**Directions:**

1. Divide the tomatoes and pierce with the skewers. Pout a little amount of olive oil in it and spray with salt and pepper.
2. Turn on the grill. On low heat, lay tomato skewer at the center of the grill.
3. Grill it for 10 minutes.
4. Prepare flatbread dough during this. Start it by cutting down the pound of dough into four equal parts. Roll every portion of dough by using flour.

Coat one side of the dough by using a pastry brush with olive oil.

5. Take tomatoes off from the grill. Put dough oil side down towards the grill. Coat the other side with oil too. Flip dough after bubbling starts to form by using a spatula. After flipping the dough, spray parmesan cheese over all the flatbreads. Take out burrata cheese from the colander. Pull small pieces off and place them smoothly on 4grilled flatbreads. Cover the lid for a few minutes to let the cheese melt. Take off flatbread from the grill & spray with basil. Serve it with tomato skewers.

**Nutrition values per serving:**
Calories: 722kcal | Proteins: 23g | Fats: 57g | Carbs: 34g

## 156. Baked Beet Chips

**Preparation time:** 5 minutes
**Cooking time:** 5 minutes
**Servings:** 4
**Ingredients:**
- 6-8 medium beets to large
- Olive oil
- 1 tbsp. flaked sea salt
- 1 tbsp. dried chives

**Directions:**
1. Trim out the green beets & roots. Scrub the beets under cold water and leave behind the skin. Use a sharp knife for slicing beets.
2. Heat the oven to 400 degrees F. Drizzle olive oil on a baking sheet pan and rub the oil over the pan using a paper towel.
3. Layer the sliced beets into the pan. Bake the chips at the bottom rack of an oven for 10 minutes, depending on how thin the beets are to cut down and how large they are.
4. While beets are baking, pour salt into a bowl. Crush the dried chives in the salt. Remove the rack and spray it with olive oil and chive salt. Allow it to cool on the pan till crisp. Repeat the process with the leftover beets.

**Nutrition values per serving:**
Calories: 55.2kcal | Proteins: 1.3g | Fats: 2.4g | Carbs: 7.8g

## 157. Smoked Salmon and Avocado Summer Rolls

**Preparation time:** 20 minutes
**Cooking time:** 0 minutes
**Servings:** 12
**Ingredients:**
- 12 round rice paper wrappers
- 6 smoked salmon slices
- 1 thinly sliced avocado
- 2-3 cups cooked vermicelli
- 1 seeded and cut into strips cucumber
- Fish sauce vinaigrette, to dip

**Directions:**
1. Take a wrapper of rice paper and submerge it into a bowl of hot tap water for 15 seconds.
2. Put the wrapper on a plate and add fillings as per your desire.
3. Fold out the bottom of the wrapper overfilling.
4. Hold the fold in place and form in a roll side.
5. Dip in the miso sesame dressing or fish sauce. Enjoy.

**Nutrition values per serving:**
Calories: 280kcal | Proteins: 24g | Fats: 11g | Carbs: 21g

## 158. Blueberry Coconut Energy Bites

**Preparation time:** 10 minutes
**Cooking time:** 10 minutes
**Servings:** 12
**Ingredients:**
- 1 cup rolled oats
- 1/4 cup ground flaxseed meal
- 2 tbsp. chia seeds
- 1/4 tsp. ground cinnamon
- Sea salt pinch
- ½ cup creamy almond butter
- ¼ cup honey
- ½ tsp. vanilla extract
- ½ tsp. coconut extract
- ¼ cup dried blueberries
- ¼ cup sweetened flaked coconut

**Directions:**
1. Mix oats, chia seeds, ground flaxseed, cinnamon, and salt in a bowl. Put almond butter in an oven and heat it for 30 seconds till smooth.
2. Add vanilla, coconut extract, and honey and mix well. Pour the oat mixture and mix it well. Stir it in the coconut & blueberries.
3. Roll the mixture into small balls. Put in an airtight container & keep refrigerated for 2 weeks.

**Nutrition values per serving:**

Calories: 165kcal | Proteins: 4g | Fats: 9g | Carbs: 19g

## 159. Izy Hossack's Falafel Smash

**Preparation time:** 10 minutes
**Cooking time:** 5 minutes
**Servings:** 4
**Ingredients:**

- 1 1/2 cups cooked chickpeas
- 1/4 tsp. salt
- 1 tsp. ground cumin
- 1 tsp. ground coriander
- 1/4 tsp. crushed red pepper
- Juice of 1/2 lemon
- 1 tbsp. olive oil
- 1/4 cup plain yogurt
- Few handfuls of pea shoots or arugula
- A pickled red onion, a few slices of thinly sliced raw red onion
- 4-6 pita bread

For cilantro sauce

- 1 garlic clove
- 2 large handfuls of cilantro
- ¼ cup olive oil
- 2 tbsp. toasted sesame seeds
- A pinch of salt

**Directions:**

1. Mash the chickpeas in a bowl with the back of a fork in a blender. Stir it in the salt, coriander, cumin, lemon juice, olive oil, and red pepper.
2. Mix all the ingredients in a bowl for the cilantro sauce.
3. Layer up the pea shoots, yogurt, arugula, cilantro sauce, chickpea mixture, and pickled on the bread & serve.

**Nutrition values per serving:**

Calories: 333kcal | Proteins: 13.3g | Fats: 17.8g | Carbs: 31.8g

## 160. Roasted Pumpkin Seeds

**Preparation time:** 10 minutes
**Cooking time:** 10 minutes
**Servings:** 3
**Ingredients:**

- 2 cups fresh pumpkin seeds
- 2 tsp. vegetable oil
- Salt & ground pepper

**Directions:**

1. Toss the pumpkin seeds with oil in a bowl. Season it with pepper and salt.
2. Add all the seeds in the basket and cook for 350 degrees and 10 minutes till crisp.

**Nutrition values per serving:**

Calories: 127kcal | Proteins: 5g | Fats: 21.4g | Carbs: 15g

## 161. Rainbow Heirloom Tomato Bruschetta

**Preparation time:** 15 minutes
**Cooking time:** 0 minutes
**Servings:** 8
**Ingredients:**

- 1 baguette
- garlic 3 cloves, halved
- 16 oz. ricotta cheese
- Kosher salt & black pepper
- ¼ cup basil pesto
- 2 tbsp. olive oil
- 2 tbsp. balsamic vinegar
- 2 tbsp. chopped dill sprigs
- 1 red tomato
- 1 halved and thinly sliced yellow tomato
- 1 halved and thinly sliced green tomato
- 1 pint heirloom cherry tomatoes
- Fresh basil leaves, for serving

**Directions:**

1. Rub the surface of each baguette slice with the garlic cloves. Season the ricotta with salt and pepper and then spread onto the baguette slices.
2. In a medium bowl, whisk together the pesto, olive oil, balsamic vinegar, and dill. Add the tomatoes and gently toss to coat. In color blocks, arrange the tomatoes on the baguette slices; season with salt and pepper. Top with basil leaves.

**Nutrition values per serving:**

Calories: 284kcal | Proteins: 12g | Fats: 15g | Carbs: 27g

# Recipes Index

## A

Artichoke & Spinach Spaghetti Squash ..... 108
Artichoke Petals Bites ..... 105
Artichoke, Chicken, and Capers with Buckwheat ..... 86
Avocado Hummus ..... 119

## B

Bagel, Jerusalem Style ..... 76
Banana Date Shakes with Tahini ..... 78
Banana Walnut Bread with Olive Oil ..... 79
Basil and Cherry Tomato Breakfast ..... 67
Bean (White) & Avocado Toast ..... 120
Bean (White) & Veggie Salad ..... 90
Beef (Stuffed) Loin in Sticky Sauce ..... 105
Beef and Veggie Salad Bowl ..... 89
Beef Cabbage Stew ..... 102
Beef Casserole, Italian Style ..... 106
Beet Chips, Baked ..... 122
Blueberry Coconut Energy Bites ..... 122
Breakfast Scramble ..... 68
Broccoli Soup, Cheesy Recipe ..... 102
Broccoli Sun-Dried Tomato Crustless Quiche ..... 67
Brussels Sprout Chips, Cheesy and Vegan ..... 119
Butternut Squash Risotto ..... 101

## C

Carrot Breakfast Salad ..... 67
Carrot Cake Energy Bites ..... 119
Carrots (Baby), Healthy Style ..... 106
Cauliflower Hash Browns ..... 72
Cauliflower Head Coated with Herbs ..... 105
Cauliflower Rice Bowls with Grilled Chicken, Greek Style ..... 110
Challah Bread ..... 75
Chicken & Avocado Salad with Grilled Lemon-Herb ..... 94
Chicken & Cucumber Greek Pita with Yogurt Sauce ..... 94
Chicken & Mango Stir Fry ..... 88
Chicken and Rice Skillet, Greek Style ..... 95
Chicken and Vegetables, Cheesy ..... 86
Chicken Breast (Grilled) with Garlic & Herbs ..... 100
Chicken Breasts (Stuffed), Mediterranean Style ..... 108
Chicken Breasts, Country Style ..... 87
Chicken Curry, African Style ..... 103
Chicken Livers with Garlic ..... 103
Chicken Merlot with Mushrooms ..... 87
Chicken Quinoa Bowl ..... 93
Chicken Salad with Stuffed Peppers and Greek Yogurt ..... 97
Chicken Shawarma, Mini ..... 96
Chicken Skewers with Tzatziki Sauce ..... 97
Chicken Skillet Pasta with Spinach, Parmesan & Lemon ..... 113
Chicken Soup, Greek Style ..... 98
Chicken Tenders, Country Style ..... 101
Chicken with Kale and Chili Sauce ..... 85
Chicken with Orzo Salad ..... 92
Chicken with Tomato-Balsamic Pan Sauce ..... 116
Chicken, Brussels Sprouts & Gnocchi, Mediterranean Style ..... 114
Chickpea Burger, Healthy Recipe ..... 104
Chickpea Quinoa Bowl, Mediterranean Style ..... 91
Chickpeas & Tuna with Mason Jar Power Salad ..... 93
Chickpeas (Roasted) with Cinnamon-Sugar ..... 119
Chickpeas with Everything-Bagel Seasoning ..... 118
Chickpeas, Buffalo Style ..... 121
Chocolate Pancakes ..... 68
Coconut Cream with Berries ..... 69
Coconut Porridge ..... 71
Couscous with Tuna & Pepperoncini, 15-Minute Recipe ..... 96
Cucumber Hummus Sandwiches ..... 120

## D

Date & Pistachio Bites (Savory) .................. 121

## E

Egg Muffins, Mediterranean Breakfast Style............. 80
Egg, Vegetarian version ................................. 79
Eggplant & Parmesan ................................... 111
Eggplant and Millet with Harissa Chickpea Stew........ 94
Eggplant, Stuffed ........................................ 99
Eggs and Veggies, Pan Baked............................ 77

## F

Falafel Smash, Izy Hossack Recipe ..................... 123
Fig & Honey Yogurt .................................... 119
Fish Curry, Thai Style ................................... 89
Flatbread (Grilled) with Burrata Cheese ................ 121
Fragrant Asian Hotpot ................................... 84
Frittata with Feta and Spinach .......................... 78
Frittata with Fresh Spinach .............................. 72
Frittata with Mozzarella, Basil, and Zucchini ........... 92
Frittata, Mediterranean Style with Veggies ............. 73
Fruit Compote, Summer Style ........................... 80

## G

Garlic Hummus ......................................... 120
Garlic Zucchini Mix ..................................... 68
Granola (Homemade) with Olive Oil and Tahini ......... 75
Green Juice, Easy Recipe ................................ 78

## H

Halloumi Cheese with Scrambled Eggs .................. 71

## K

Kale Chips ............................................... 118

## L

Lamb Curry ............................................. 106
Lamb, Butternut Squash, and Date Tagine ............... 83
Lamb, Mediterranean Style ............................. 104
Lemon Bars ............................................. 116
Lentil Soup, Vegan Mediterranean Recipe .............. 111

## M

Meatball Mezze Bowls, Greek Style ..................... 90
Mushroom (Portobello) Pizzas with Arugula Salad ... 107
Mushrooms & Peppers (Stuffed), Easy Breakfast ....... 81
Mushrooms (Portobello ), Caprese ..................... 114
Mushrooms with Camembert ........................... 106

## O

Oatmeal ................................................. 69
Omelet with Mushroom ................................. 71
Omelet with Seafood ................................... 69
Omelet, Chili Style ...................................... 73
Omelet, Loaded Mediterranean Style ................... 82
Omelet, Persian Style (Kuku Sabzi ) .................... 82
Omelet, Western Style .................................. 71

## P

Peanut Butter Energy Balls ............................. 118
Pesto Chicken Salad with Greens ....................... 93
Pesto Eggs with Tomato and Mozzarella ............... 74
Pesto Quinoa Bowls with Roasted Veggies and
    Labneh ............................................... 97
Pistachio & Peach Toast ................................ 121
Pistachio-Crusted Salmon with Broccoli ................ 117
Prawn (King) with Buckwheat Noodles ................. 84
Prawn Arrabbiata ....................................... 85
Prosciutto Pizza with Corn & Arugula .................. 110
Pumpkin Bread, Spicy ................................... 70
Pumpkin Greek Yogurt Parfait, 5-minute Recipe ....... 79
Pumpkin Seeds, Roasted ............................... 123

## Q

Quinoa Bowls, Mediterranean Style .......................... 98
Quinoa Protein Bars ................................................ 104
Quinoa with Arugula, Mediterranean Style ............. 107
Quinoa, Avocado & Chickpea Salad over Mixed Greens ................................................................. 113

## R

Raspberry Clafoutis .................................................. 77
Ravioli with Artichokes & Olives, Mediterranean Style ................................................................... 109

## S

Salad Skewers ........................................................... 85
Salmon (Baked) Salad with Mint Dressing ................ 83
Salmon (Roasted, Sweet & Spicy) with Wild Rice Pilaf ............................................................. 114
Salmon (Seared) with Braised Broccoli ..................... 89
**Salmon (Smoked) and Avocado Summer Rolls** ...... 122
Salmon Filled Avocado .............................................. 72
Salmon with Fennel & Sun-Dried Tomato Couscous ............................................................ 113
Salmon with Sweet Potatoes & Broccoli ................. 109
Salmon, Smoked ....................................................... 75
Scrambled Eggs with Tomatoes, Turkish Style ......... 74
Sesame-Crusted Mahi-Mahi ................................... 100
Shakshuka with Spinach, Chard & Feta .................. 112
Shakshuka, Classic Recipe ........................................ 77
Shakshuka, Green Recipe ......................................... 76
Shrimp (Charred), Pesto & Quinoa Bowls ............... 109
Shrimp B.B.Q. Style with Garlicky Kale & Parmesan-Herb Couscous .................................. 112
Shrimp Deviled Eggs ................................................. 70
Shrimp, Cajun Style ................................................ 100

Spinach & Egg Scramble with Raspberries ................ 92
Spinach and Pork with Fried Eggs ............................. 70
Stew, Mediterranean Recipe (Slow-Cooker ) ........... 110
Strawberry & Cherry Smoothie ................................. 73

## T

Tacos (Mahi-Mahi) with Avocado and Fresh Cabbage ............................................................. 101
Tilapia with Wilted Greens & Mushrooms, Mediterranean Style .......................................... 115
Tilapia, Fried ........................................................... 102
Toast, Mediterranean-Style Breakfast ...................... 80
Tomato (Heirloom) and Cucumber Toast ................. 95
Tomato (Heirloom) Bruschetta .............................. 123
Tomato, Cucumber & White-Bean Salad with Basil Vinaigrette ............................................... 91
Tomato-Basil Skewers ............................................ 120
Tuna and Kale ........................................................... 88
Tuna and Spinach Salad ............................................ 91
Tuna Casserole with Buckwheat ............................... 86
Turkey Lettuce Wraps ............................................... 90
Turkey with Capers, Tomatoes, and Greens Beans ... 89
Turkey with Cauliflower Couscous ........................... 88

## W

Walnut-Rosemary Crusted Salmon .......................... 107

## Z

Za'atar Olive Oil Fried Eggs ...................................... 73
Zoodles Salad ........................................................... 98
Zucchini Crustless Quiche ........................................ 81
Zucchini Lasagna Rolls with Smoked Mozzarella .... 115
Zucchini Omelet ....................................................... 67

BONUS CHAPTER

# 7-DAY Workout PLAN

## Easy to Follow Exercises to Boost the Benefits of Intermittent Fasting

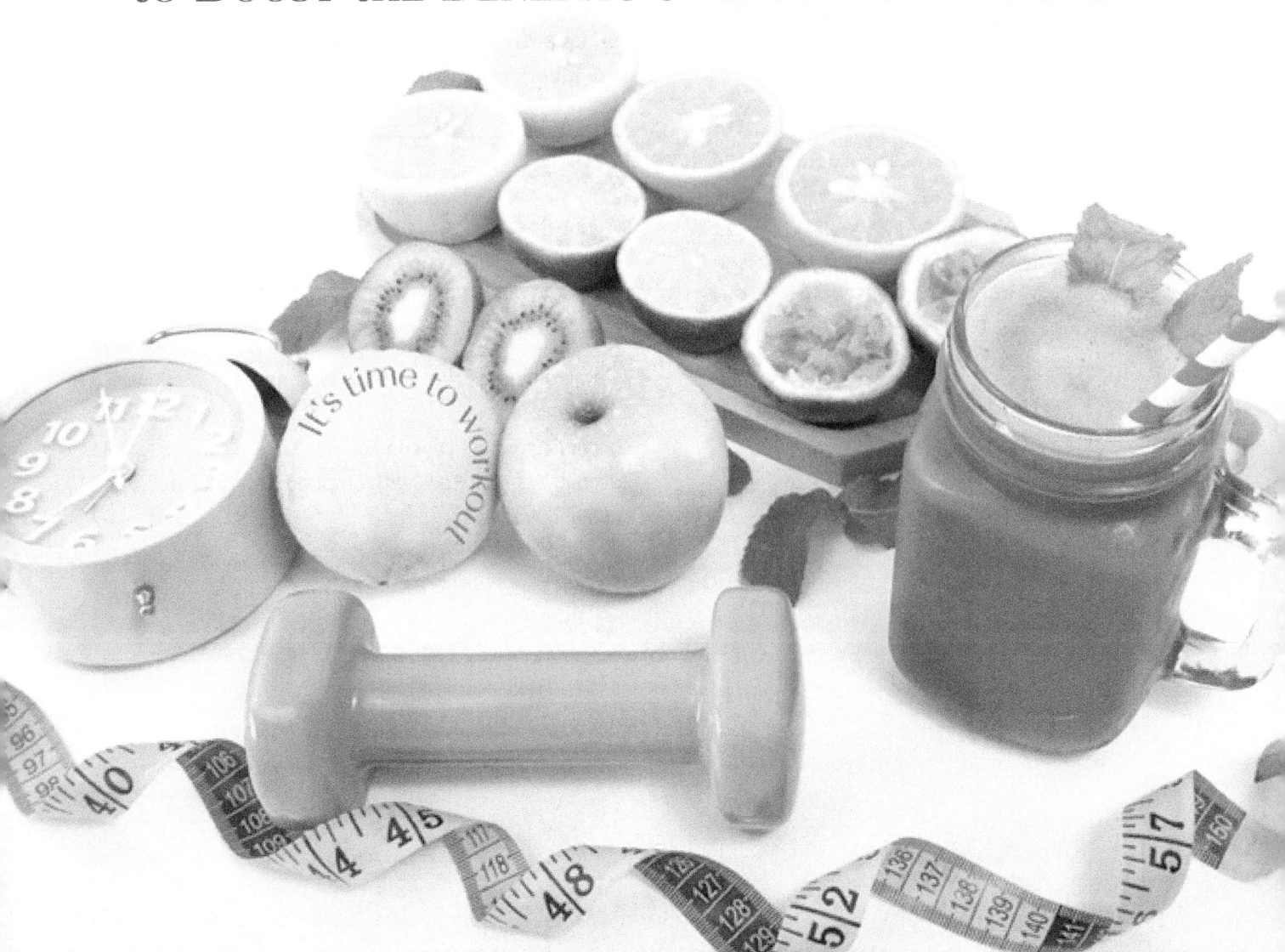

# Day 1

## Day 1 - WARMUP

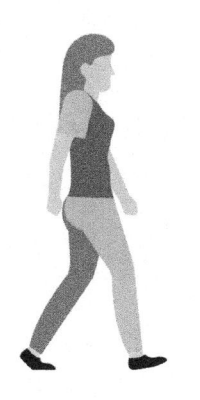

### WALKING | 10 Minutes

Walking is the simplest workout strategy, especially for the senior population of the '50s. Walk helps in making the heart-healthy. Moreover, it lowers blood pressure, makes the bones strong, and increases muscle mass. Walking will not target the core of the body. It will not affect the arms. The major impact of walking is on the muscles of the lower limb. Walking exercise does not cause any impact on the back muscles. It mostly increases the strength of leg muscles and makes them strong and volumetrically massive

## Day 1 - ARMS

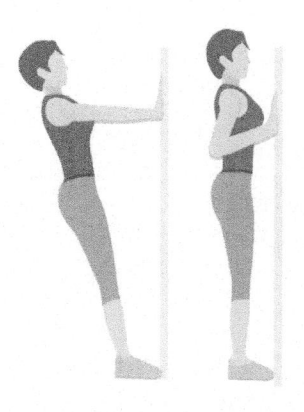

### WALL PUSH-UPS | 2 Sets x 10 Repetitions

This exercise mainly focuses on the fitness and strength of the triceps muscles. Stand straight, put the hand on the wall and stretch the arms. Try to push the wall away by putting the complete body weight over the arms. Repeat 10 times per 2 sets

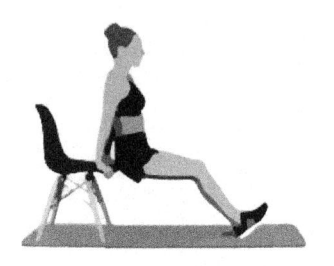

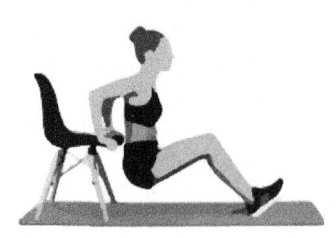

### BENCH DIPS | 10 Repetition

The main target is the bicep and triceps muscle. Sit on a chair. Put the hands on the bench in a comfortable position. Now leave the bench and bend on the knees keeping the whole burden on the arms' muscles. Push the back up and repeat the step 10 times. If at the beginning you can't do the exercise, simply sit on the floor with your legs stretched out and try to lift your glutes by placing your hands next to your hips and extending your arms

## Day 1 – STRETCHING

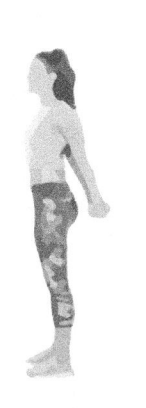

### ARM OPENER | 5 Sets x 20-30 Secs

The Arm opener helps to stretch the chest, arms, and shoulders. To do this exercise, stand straight with both feet at a distance of a few inches. Now, interlace both your hands after taking them behind your back. Keep the palms in a downwards direction. Keep your face and back as straight as possible. Then, slowly move your arms up and down and try to keep your hands away from your back. This will stretch your arms a little. While doing the exercise, take deep breaths to support your respiratory system. Hold for 20 to 30 seconds before relaxing

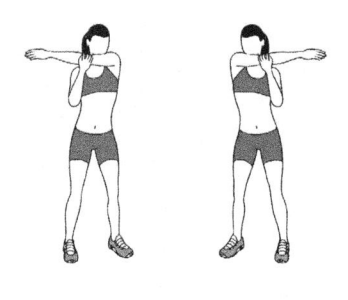

### SHOULDER STRETCH | 5 Repetitions

Cross one arm over your chest and keep it straight. With the opposite arm, grasp the elbow and gently draw it toward your chest. Hold for 10 to 20 seconds before repeating on the other side. This is 1 repetition

# Day 2

## Day 2 - WARMUP

### WALKING | 15 Minutes

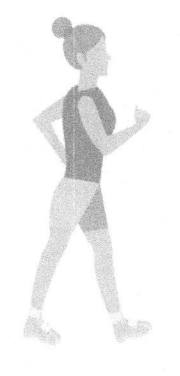

Do 15 minutes of the casual slow walk as a warmup. Where you find stairs, if you are outside, try to climb up and down 3-4 times. Otherwise you can try to speed up the walk the last 5 minutes

## Day 2 – LEGS

### STEP UP | 2 Sets x 10 Repetitions

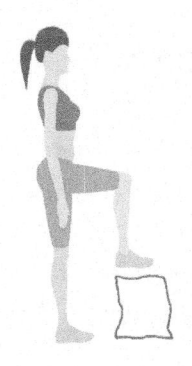

Put a step platform (or similar) in your front about 1 foot away, step up the left foot and drive the right knee up in the direction of the chest. Now take the right leg towards the starting position. This is the 1st repetition

*Healthy Recipes*

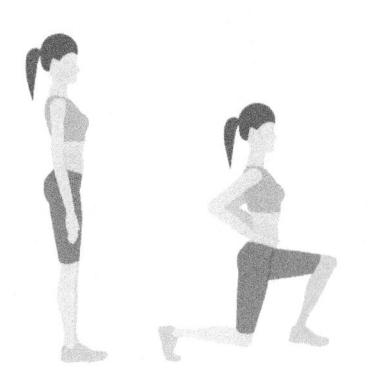

### REVERSE LUNGE | 2 Sets x 5 Repetitions

Take a standing position; take the left leg backward while inhaling, hold the position for 5-10 seconds and then take the leg back to the starting position. Repeat the step for the second leg. This is 1 repetition

### PILE SQUAT | 2 Sets x 5 Repetitions

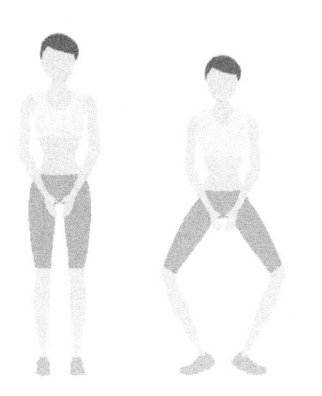

Take a standing position, widen the legs keeping the arms on the thighs and toes outwards. Bend on the knees and hold the position for a minimum of 10 seconds. Repeat the exercise 10 times

## Day 2 – STRETCHING

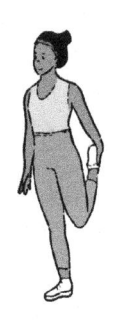

### QUAD STRETCH | 5 Repetitions x 30 Secs

Stand with your feet hip-width apart. While standing on your right leg, grip your left ankle with your left hand and lift your foot to meet your buttocks (you should feel the stretch in the front of your thigh). Hold for up to 30 seconds and then switch the leg. This is 1 repetition.
This practice is another way to teach you to balance one leg while also stretching out your quadriceps

## CALF STRETCHE | 5 Repetitions x 30 Secs

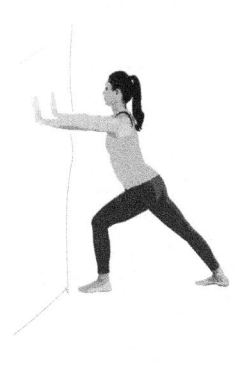

To keep your balance, keep an arm's length away from a wall or a desk. Put your right foot behind your left. Lean forward slowly toward the wall or desk while maintaining your right heel flat on the floor. Make an effort to maintain your back straight. Bend your knee as you travel forward for a deeper stretch. Hold for 30 seconds and then change the leg. This is 1 Repetition

# Day 3

## Day 3 – WARMUP & CARDIO

### WALKING | 5 Minutes

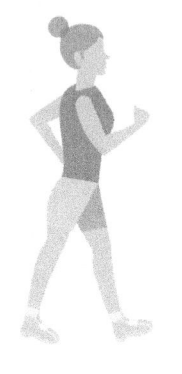

Do 5 minutes of the casual slow walk as a warmup. Try to walk a bit faster than your normal walk

### SLOW FROGGER | 2 Sets x 10 Repetitions

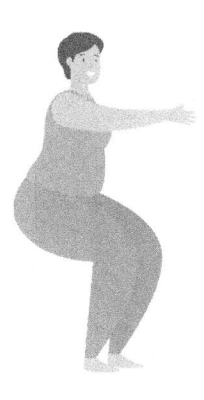

Take a straight position on the mat and slightly bend on the knees. Wide the legs and join both hands, pointing upwards straight in the direction of eyes. Now try to take a slight jump. Repeat the process 10 times per 2 Sets, taking at least 1 minute rest in between the sets

# Day 3 – ABS & CORE

### CORE STABILIZER | 10 Repetition x 3 Sets

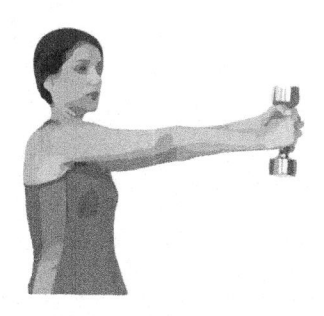

Stand straight on the mat. Keep the body stretched and hold a dumbbell in the hands (or other equal weights). Take the dumbbell straight in the front of the chest. Now slightly move the torso and rotate the arms first in the right direction and then in the left. Hold one position for 10 seconds and then take the next position. Repeat the exercise 10 times per 3 sets

### OBLIQUE BEND | 10 Repetition x 2 Sets

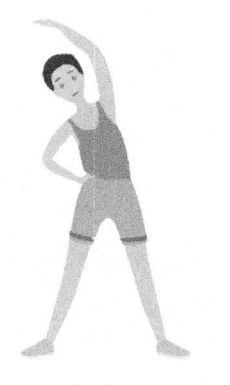

Take a straight position on the floor and keep the arms stretched. Put one hand on the side and take the other hand stretched in the opposite direction while bending slightly. Repeat the process for the other side as well. Hold one position for 15 seconds. Repeat the exercise 10 times per side per 2 sets

# Day 3 – STRETCHING

### HULA HOOP | 5 Minutes

This exercise helps stretch your legs and hips, allowing you to keep your lower body in an active and flexible state. To do this exercise, stand straight with hands holding your waist. Then move your waist in clockwise and anticlockwise directions without moving your upper body parts. While doing this stretching exercise, keep your back and shoulders straight, and your stomach pulled in

## NECK STRETCH | 3 Sets x 5 cycles

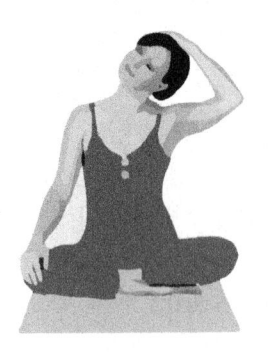

Sit on the edge of a yoga mat or a rug. Extend your legs in front of you, sit up straight, and then insert each foot under the opposite knee. Try to distribute your weight equally over your sit bones. Align your head, neck, and spine. Lengthen your spine while softening your neck. On your next breath, softly lower your right ear toward your right shoulder. Inhale as you return your head to the center. Exhale once more as you lower your left ear toward your left shoulder. Repeat this cycle five times, then return your head to the center.
Lean back and alter the cross of your legs

## CHIN DROP | 10 Repetitions

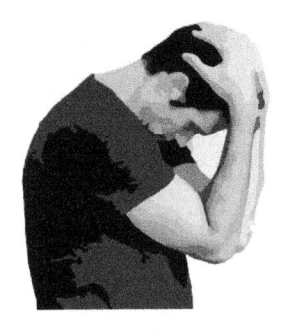

This helps to stretch your shoulders and neck. Sit in a comfortable place and position with your back straight. Now bring your elbows in front of you. Bend your head and hold it with your hands. With the help of the strength of your arms, put pressure on your head in a downwards direction so that you may feel a stretch in your shoulders and neck. Inhale and exhale ten times and repeat the process 10 times

# Day 4

## Day 4 – WARMUP

### WALKING | 15 Minutes

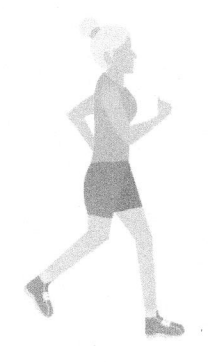

Do 15 minutes of the casual slow walk as a warmup. Where you find stairs, if you are outside, try to climb up and down 3-4 times. Otherwise, you can try to speed up the walk the last 5 minutes

## Day 4 – LEGS & GLUTES

### SPLIT SQUAT | 2 Sets x 5 Repetitions

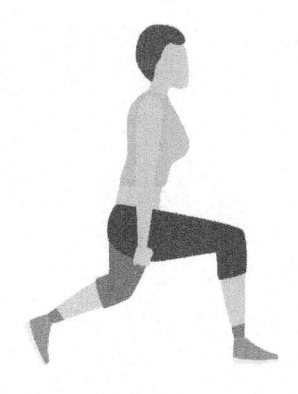

Sit down in a straight position on the weight of toes. Take one foot forward in front of the other. Stretch the shoulders back. Place the hand on thighs and hold this position for 10-15 seconds. Repeat the process with the second leg. This is 1 repetition

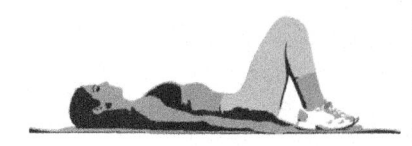

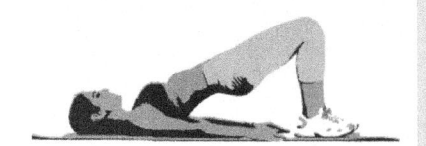

### GLUTES BRIDGE | 2 Sets x 10 Repetitions

Lie down straight on the floor and lift the but by putting the whole burden on the leg muscles. Place the arms on the floor and take the support of arms to lift the body. Hold the position for 10-15 seconds. Repeat the process 10 times per 2 sets

## Day 4 – STRETCHING

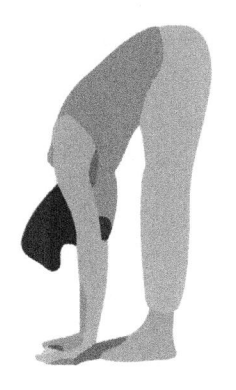

### FORWARD BEND | 10 Repetitions x 20 Secs

Stand straight on the floor. Take the arms up and bend on the knees. Bend the arms such that the palms of the hands touch the floor. Hold the position for 15-20 seconds. Repeat 10 times

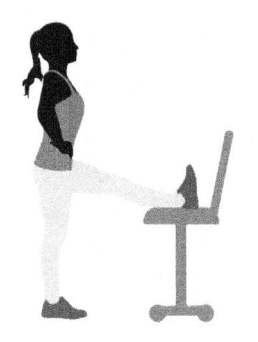

### STANDING HAMSTRING STRETCH | 10 Repetitions x 30 Secs

Place one foot on a low table, chair, or stair step. Bend forward from your hips while standing tall, maintaining your chest high, hips square, and tailbone raised. You should now feel a stretch at the back of your leg or knee. Stretch for 20-30 seconds and then repeat with the opposing leg

# Day 5

## Day 5 – WARMUP

### WALKING | 10 Minutes

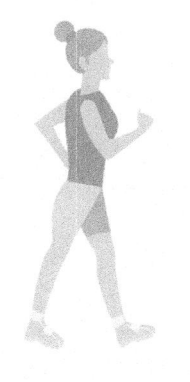

First, take a warmup round for 5 through a slow walk and light jumps like row skipping, and then start brisk walking for 10 minutes

## Day 5 - ARMS

### CROSSOVER JUMPING JACKS | 15 Repetition x 2 Sets

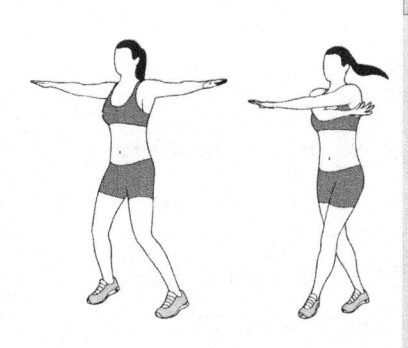

Stand with your feet shoulder-width apart and your arms straight out to either side, palms down. This is your starting point. Cross your right arm over your left arm and your right foot over your left foot as you jump. Return to your starting posture and cross with the opposing arm and foot. This counts as one repetition. Alternate sides and continue this action until you have completed 25 repetitions. Keep the tempo up, and don't take too much time (if you feel ok) to recuperate between leaps; this way, you'll be sure to keep your heart rate up and utilize your whole body

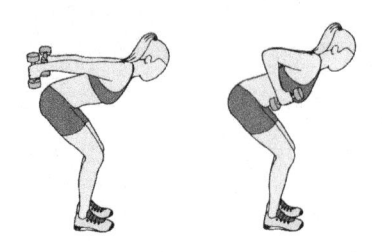

## TRICEPS KICKBACK | 15 Repetition x 2 Sets

To do this, sit on a bench or in any comfortable position. Hold the light dumbbells in hand and slightly bend forward. Now move the arms in a backward position and slightly give a stretched jerk. Repeat the process 15 times per 2 sets. In the beginning, you may not use any weight

# Day 5 – STRETCHING

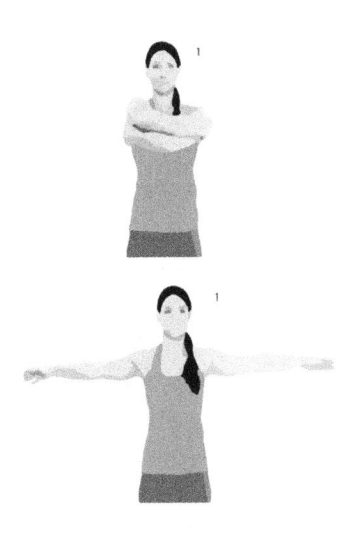

## BEAR HUG | 10 Repetitions x 20 Secs

This stretching mainly works on the trapezius muscles of the upper body. It helps to relieve the pain due to some poor posture. Stand up and take a straight position. First, stretch the arms and then make a cross while exhaling. Hold this stretch position for 20 seconds. Repeat the process 10 times

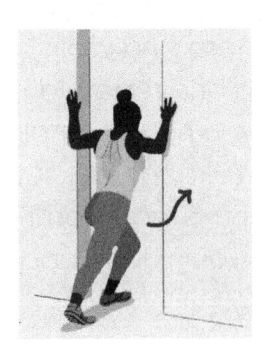

## DOORWAY PECTORAL STRETCH | 40 Sec. x 5 Times

This is to stretch your chest and shoulders. Open the door and stand straight in the doorway. Now, lift your arms and place them on the sides of the doorway (arms should be at ninety degrees). Move your one leg forward; this will put some pressure on your shoulders. Keep this position for 40 seconds and repeat the process 5 times

# Day 6

## Day 6 – WARMUP

### WALKING | 10 Minutes

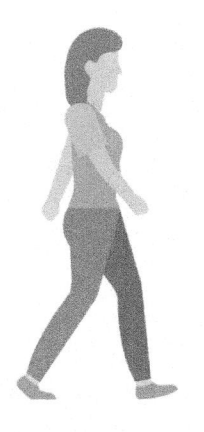

Do 10 minutes of the casual slow walk as a warmup. Where you find stairs, if you are outside, try to climb up and down 3-4 times. Otherwise, you can try to speed up the walk the last 5 minutes

## Day 6 – ABS & CORE

### MARCH WITH A TWIST | 10 minutes

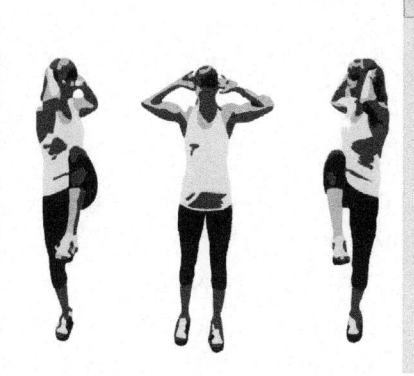

Stand straight with the hands and legs apart. Keep the arms apart upward, lift the right leg, and try to touch the knee with the elbow of the left arm, similarly, for the opposite. Repeat the exercise for 10 minutes

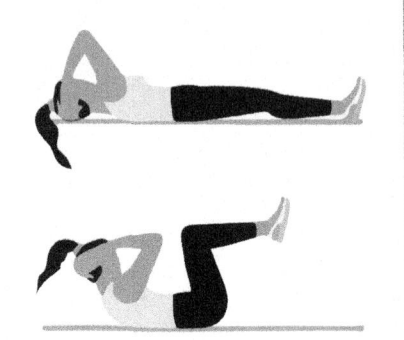

### KNEE-IN CRUNCH | 3 Sets x 5 Repetitions

Lie faceup with your hands behind your ears and your legs outstretched. Raise your legs until your feet are approximately 6 inches above the floor. Engage your core and raise your shoulder blades off the floor. Come up like and draw your knees in toward your chest. Take care not to strain your neck by lifting with your abs. To return to the initial position, reverse the movement

## Day 6 – STRETCHING & POSTURE

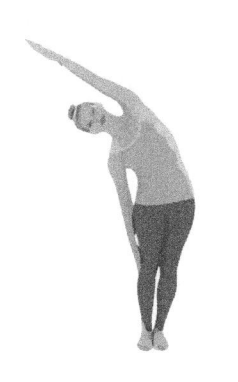

### STANDING SIDE BEND | 2 Repetitions

This exercise is to improve your posture and stretch your oblique and spine. For this exercise, stand straight with both the feet touching each other and both arms at your side touching your body. Now move your left arm upwards in a straight line. Bend yourself a little in the opposite direction of the straight arm. Inhale and exhale at this position ten times and repeat the process to the opposite side with the right arm. This is 1 repetition

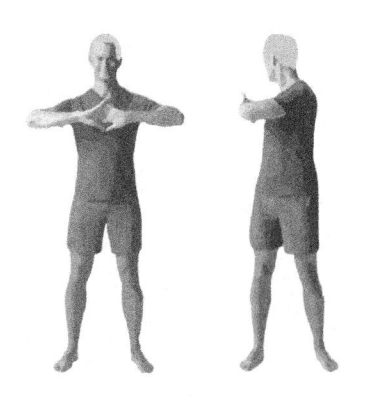

### YO-YO STRETCH | 3 cycles

Yo-yo stretch exercise is for posture and spine. For yo-yo stretch, stand straight on your feet, feet at the distance of 5 inches. Toes should be in the outwards direction. Now, interlock your hands in such a way that your palm is facing away from you, and they are in front of your chest with elbows straight. Then, slightly twist your shoulders with elbows in a clockwise and anticlockwise direction. Stretch in both directions, 5 times, as much as you can. This is 1 cycle. Remember to start with a little stretching and slowly increase the stretch after a few times. Try to keep your lower body at rest to gain maximum outcomes

# Day 7

## Day 7 – WARMUP

### WALKING and JUMPING | 5 Minutes

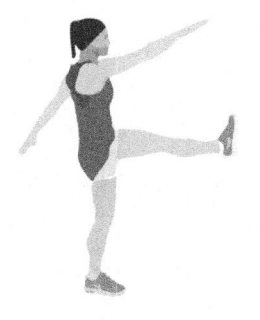

Take a warmup round through slight jumping and stretching. It will relax the body and increase the blood flow

## Day 7 – BALANCE

### IN-PLACE MARCHES | 2 Sets x 5 Minutes

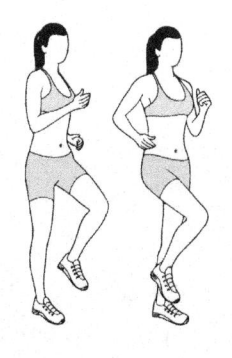

To do this, 1st stretch the arms outwards. Look straight forward and keep the chin straight. Now place one foot in front of the other foot and walk. Do this for 5 minutes per 2 times

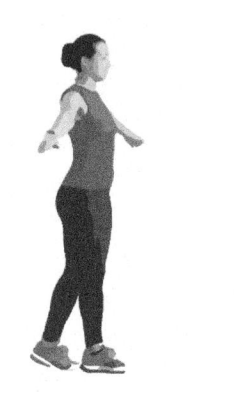

## HEEL TO TOE WALK | 10 Minutes

It is such a balance training workout that can be done indoors. It is effective and mostly recommended for all age groups. To do this, 1st stretch the arms outwards and look straight forward and keep the chin straight. Now place one foot in front of the other foot and walk. Do this for 10 minutes

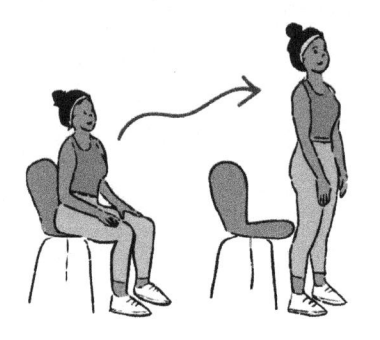

## CHAIR SITS | 5 Repetitions

Stand with your back against a chair and your feet hip-width apart. Slowly drop your hips into the chair and wait for a second before sitting. Then, push through your heels to get back to standing. Do this ten times, which is 1 repetition. If this exercise seems to be almost absurdly easy, that's because it is. When it comes to developing balance, often the simplest motions are the most beneficial

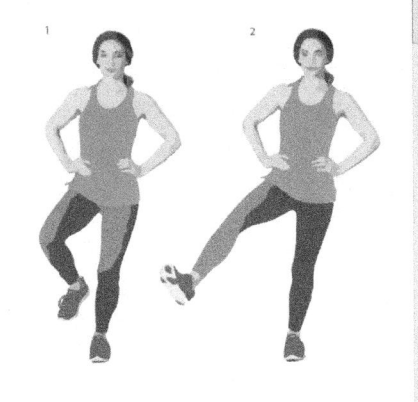

## BALANCE | 5 Repetitions

Stand with the feet and hip-width apart. Put the hands on the sides and lift one leg. Hold the position for 10 seconds and repeat the process 10 times. Same for the second leg. This is 1 repetition

# Conclusion

Intermittent Fasting has become popular in Western countries. It is defined as a dietary regimen where you fast intermittently by going without food or caloric beverages for an extended period of time. This can be for as short as 12 hours and up to 21 days.

The most common variations are a) fasting for 14–16 hours and b) fasting every second day for 24 hours. The latter is also known as "the 5:2 diet" because people on this schedule normally eat 5 days a week, with their calorie intake being "capped" at 600–700 calories (on fasting days), and then eating just 500 calories 2 days of the week.

The rise of Intermittent Fasting has led to a plethora of spin-offs, including the 5:2 diet, which I'll refer to as the "5:2 plan" from now on. This includes improvements in body composition, insulin sensitivity, triglycerides, and cholesterol. These studies are limited by their small sample sizes (typically less than 20 participants), and typically use a short-term intervention strategy (e.g., 11 days) with a limited time frame (e.g., 24 hours).

In the context of Intermittent Fasting, some individuals tend to go overboard on their calorie "capping." For example, they might cut out all food or drink for 24 hours every second day while attempting to eat as much as possible on fast days. This isn't recommended for 2 reasons: first of all, it is too difficult to maintain such a strict diet because almost everything you eat or drink contains calories which will take up those calories on the fasting days. Secondly, this approach may lead to undesirable physiological adaptations as the body's metabolism tends to adapt in an attempt to preserve energy.

To sum up, Intermittent Fasting is a popular dietary intervention used by many people for various reasons, and there are no strong indications that it is harmful. In the event that you haven't set any well-being and health objectives with the data you have learned here, your following stage is to do as such!

Intermittent Fasting isn't just a weight reduction diet methodology. It implies far more than that. It has a few well-being and health benefits that won't simply make you slimmer, a lot better, and sickness-free. There is comparably a great deal of determinations that accompany Intermittent Fasting, so you can pick the choice that will work the very best for you. Intermittent fasting is key, easy to work with, and furthermore, viable.

At the point when you are prepared to decrease weight or improve your well-being and health, allude back to this manual to help you take off. IF gives incredible arrangements of advantages to your body. Regardless of whether you intend to diminish weight or improve your health, Intermittent Fasting is the best approach.

Having said that, I wish you to have fabulous years after the 50s!

Made in the USA
Monee, IL
20 December 2021